To all those women—mothers, aunts, sisters, cousins, friends—who are approaching the dawn of a new phase in life

Before the Change

ALSO BY
ANN LOUISE GITTLEMAN, M.S., C.N.S.

The 40/30/30 Phenomenon

Get the Salt Out

Get the Sugar Out

Your Body Knows Best

Beyond Pritikin

Super Nutrition for Men

Super Nutrition for Women

Super Nutrition for Menopause

Guess What Came to Dinner

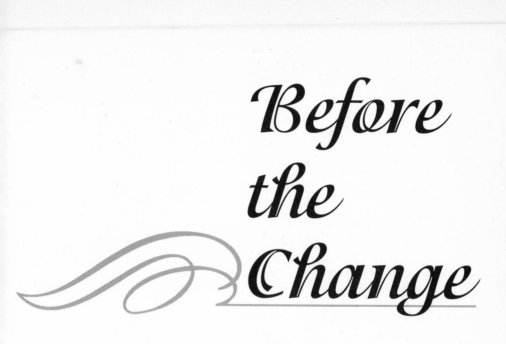

Before the Change

Taking Charge of Your Perimenopause

Ann Louise Gittleman, M.S., C.N.S.

HarperSanFrancisco

A Division of HarperCollins*Publishers*

HarperCollins Web Site: http://www.harpercollins.com

HarperCollins®, ⚑ ®, and HarperSanFrancisco™ are
trademarks of HarperCollins Publishers Inc.

FIRST EDITION

Library of Congress Cataloging-in-Publication Data

Gittleman, Ann Louise
    Before the change: Taking charge of your perimenopause /
Ann Louise Gittleman.
        p. cm.
    Includes bibliographical references and index.
    ISBN 0-06-251539-X (cloth)
    ISBN 0-06-251537-3 (pbk.)
    1. Menopause—Popular works. 2. Menopause—
Complications—Diet therapy. 3. Middle aged women—
Nutrition. I. Title.
RG186.G568 1997
618.1'75—dc21   97-32146

98 99 00 01 02 RRD(H) 10 9 8 7 6 5 4 3 2 1

Contents

Acknowledgments

I would like to acknowledge the assistance and patience of my editor, Caroline Pincus, and her assistant, Sally Kim. Also at my publisher, I would like to thank Margery Buchanan, Amy Durgan, Alisa Ikeda, Terri Leonard, Meg Lenihan, Karen Bouris, Lisa Zuniga, and Priscilla Stuckey. Thanks to George Ryan for his creative mastery, and to my agent and good friend Michael Cohn.

American women today owe much to the pioneering work in female health of Drs. John Lee, Christiane Northrup, and Jonathan Wright. I have benefitted greatly from their expertise, and from that of Drs. Ray Sahelian, Stephen Langer, Leo Frangipane, Julian Whitaker, Joan Borysenko, Caroline Myss, Norman Shealy, Ronald Hoffman, Robert Atkins, Cass Igram, Sydney Baker, and Jacob Teitelbaum. As well as being of assistance to me, their work has been a great inspiration.

I would like to express appreciation for the help given to me by Stuart and Sandra Gittleman, Marilyn Caine, and Marie Lugano. A special acknowledgment needs to be made to all those women who have been my supporters and helpers in so many ways, notably including Joyce Piersanti, Dianna Frederick, Cheryl Miller, Christine Nilsson, Cheryl Townsley, Marcia Smith, Gillian D'Armond, Jane Heimlich, Phyllis Herman, Denise Silvestro, Deborah Ray, Danielle Lin, Charlotte Norrie, Joanie Greggains, Cindy Renshaw, Ann Wixon, Monica Reinagel, Jolie Martin Root, Vicki Accardi, Melissa Diane Smith, Beth Salmon, Karolyn Gazella, and Kathryn Arnold. Special thanks to my treasured companion and colleague, James William Templeton.

I hope that, in reading this book, you will recognize the gratitude I feel toward all the women who have shared information with me about their perimenopausal symptoms, challenges and triumphs.

Foreword

It's not exactly polite to congratulate a woman on her age, but if such congratulations are coupled with compliments on her wisdom, one just might get by.

Readers of this book have every reason to be grateful that Ann Louise Gittleman is the age she is. Were she considerably younger, she would not have suffered insomnia, palpitations, irritability, impatience, and many other discomforts of perimenopause, that time of a woman's life prior to menopause when menstrual periods are occurring but hormone levels are declining. She would not have had the motivation to find out what was happening to her.

But motivation is only one part of what it took. Ann Louise is to be congratulated even more on her wisdom and just plain common sense in deciding that her symptoms were not "all in her head" but were real physical symptoms with physical causes. She then set out on a journey of discovery to find out not only what those causes were but what could be done to prevent and treat them.

Ann Louise is one of the leaders in the "natural health care revolution," a leader who writes and teaches self-care through safe, effective, natural means. As she has explained in her previous books and articles, our bodies are natural systems living in a natural world, nourished and kept healthy by natural means. When symptoms occur, they frequently signal malfunctions in our natural living systems that can be corrected and prevented by natural means, if we can only discover what those means are.

Which brings us to another "Congratulations!" to Ann Louise on her wisdom: as the pages that follow clearly demonstrate, she has figured out many of the reasons why she and other women develop perimenopausal symptoms and what can be done to prevent them or to eliminate them if they occur.

By definition, perimenopausal symptoms are due to declining, fluctuating sex hormone levels. Most of us, including many doctors, have thought of sex hormones mostly in terms of, well, sex, and the obviously related subjects of sexual organs, babies, and so on. But in recent years, researchers have discovered "sex hormone receptors" (locations on cell membranes specifically designed to receive sex hormones and transmit their "messages" into the cell) on nearly every cell in our bodies. Estrogen, progesterone, and other hormones of the menstrual cycle are not just "female sex hormones" with the limited purposes of growing breasts, hips, and babies. There are estrogen receptors on brain cells, progesterone receptors on bones, receptors for both on white cells, receptors for estrogen and progesterone nearly everywhere!

Research at Columbia University has shown that maintaining estrogen levels after the menopause can prevent a significant proportion of senility, certainly a "non-sex-related" effect of estrogens. If estrogens after the menopause can prevent senility, then certainly stabilizing and maintaining estrogen levels "before the change" can have a favorable effect on mental health. At Tahoma Clinic, we've observed the effect of natural progesterone in actually rebuilding thinned-out, osteoporotic bones for women over 60, another "non-sex-related" effect of a "sex hormone." (This observation was first made by Dr. John Lee of Sebastopol, California.) It just makes sense that if we can better stabilize and maintain progesterone levels "before the change," we can have stronger bones for a longer time, and worry less about osteoporosis after menopause.

The marked decline of estrogens and progesterone at menopause can lead to increased risk of senility, osteoporosis, atherosclerosis, and generally accelerated aging of nearly every part of a woman's body. It just makes logical sense that the slow, subtle decline of these same hormones prior to the menopause will also cause slow, subtle (and, in some cases, not so subtle) disruptions of function nearly everywhere in her body. But if these disruptions lead to symptoms serious enough for her to visit a doctor, no disease will be found, as perimenopause isn't a disease. She'll be told "It's just your age" or "It's stress, just relax" or the ever-popular "It's all in your head." She may be prescribed a tranquilizer or some other symptom-relieving drug.

In one sense, the doctor is correct. Perimenopausal symptoms are not due to disease; perimenopause is a time of life. But it's a time of life to be enjoyed as much as any other, and not a time to be troubled, slightly or greatly, with the unnecessary distraction of a malfunctioning body. Thanks to Ann Louise's wisdom, hard work, and (sorry about that, Ann Louise) age, readers of this book can prevent and, if necessary, correct any symptoms of the perimenopause with safe, effective, nondrug, natural means, and get on with experiencing and enjoying this time of life.

Now that age has come up again, why not mention mine? (I'll admit to being older than Ann Louise.) After medical school graduation in 1969, I prescribed synthetic and other unnatural hormones for women in menopause just as I'd been taught. Fortunately, I learned what Ann Louise knows and teaches, that it's best to use natural means for our natural bodies whenever possible. Since 1982 I've prescribed natural hormones identical to the ones present in a woman's body "before the change." Women using natural hormones have felt considerably better than they did with the various synthetics and have less risk of adverse effects. Very recently I've written a book about natural hormone replacement.

In her last chapter, Ann Louise writes about hormone replacement "after the change" and shares her first "hot flash" with us, a hot flash experienced as she was reading about hot flashes! She briefly discusses hormone replacement—synthetic, unnatural, and natural—and advises, as she does throughout the rest of the book, that natural means are best and safest. Once again, congratulations to Ann Louise for her wisdom, and many thanks for putting so much of it in this book.

Jonathan V. Wright, M.D.
Medical Director, Tahoma Clinic
Kent, Washington

Part 1

Alleviating Symptoms

Chapter 1

Peri-what?

What on earth was happening to my body? Exhausted after several nights of not being able to sleep properly, here I was again, awake at 4 A.M., feeling palpitations in my heart. Until this began, I would have slept through a hurricane. Was this the start of a heart condition or a nervous breakdown?

After a productive but extremely stressful year of travel, radio shows, lectures, and book promotions, I had relocated my office and was in the midst of remodeling my home. While the pressure of all these activities had propelled me to a new level of stress and tension, I kept reminding myself that in the past I had thrived under pressure. Anyway, no matter how much stress I had been under—from manuscript deadlines to speeches in front of thousands of people—once my head hit that pillow, I was out and always slept through the night.

Something was definitely changing in my body. I began to imagine the possibility of never getting a good night's sleep again, and that made me feel even more anxious and depressed.

It wasn't until I took an entire battery of blood tests (including an FSH hormone indicator) that it dawned on me what was really happening. At age forty-plus, I was in perimenopause. My concept of perimenopause was academic. But I knew that it was a time of about ten years in a woman's life during which her body changes its secretion and processing of the hormones needed for reproduction. Two months earlier, for the first time in my life I had missed a period, but I'd attributed it to excessive travel and the body clock adjustments that come with flying through various time zones.

Yet it was also true that over the past ten years I had become noticeably more irritable and less patient—with a shorter fuse—and had developed a shorter attention span. I simply attributed these personality changes to my increased focus on work. It never once occurred to me that something biochemical, such as hormones, was changing in my body, affecting my nervous system. Additionally, I didn't have any telltale symptoms like hot flashes or night sweats.

Now I realized that if only I had recognized what was happening to me, I would have sought remedies much earlier on. Those ten years could have been far more pleasurable for me than they were. I say this even though my symptoms were not as severe as those suffered by many women during their perimenopause.

Motivated by my own experience, I set out on a mission to enlighten women everywhere, between the ages of thirty-five and fifty, about this newly recognized stage of life called perimenopause. In addition to comparing notes with women from this age group all over the country, I attended perimenopause conferences, reviewed special publications, and interviewed doctors, psychologists, researchers, and product developers. I also personally experimented with a variety of remedies based upon state-of-the-art comprehensive hormone profiles.

What I learned was appalling. The scant information available on perimenopause was frequently incomplete, misleading, and highly risky to follow. American women are being told to take tranquilizers for nervousness and anxiety and sleeping pills for disturbed sleeping patterns—symptoms caused by the hormonal imbalances of perimenopause. The use of the antidepressant

Prozac, a much-recommended drug for a number of female symptoms, is up 65.4 percent in just the last three years, with 18 million prescriptions written.

Millions of women never discover the fundamental cause of their emotional and physical symptoms. As menopause specialist Dr. Helene B. Leonetti states, "I would say that 50 percent of women in perimenopause have been misdiagnosed. Usually they've been given Prozac or put through a ten-thousand-dollar cardiac workup." Dr. Nancy Lee Teaff, author of *Perimenopause: Preparing for the Change,* told *New Woman* magazine: "When they first start to appear, perimenopausal symptoms may seem unrelated to each other, and women often treat each problem individually, not seeing the connection until years later." She continued, "Skipped periods and hot flashes are almost automatically attributed to menopause, but if your first symptom happens to be insomnia, you may spend hours in a therapist's office before it becomes apparent that the problem is primarily hormonal."

Women desperately seek new remedies for fresh symptoms, but they look in all the wrong places! They try to treat each symptom as a separate problem, while instead they need to discover the single underlying cause. Once they restore greater balance to their hormones, their symptoms usually fade and may disappear on their own. But to do this, a woman has to recognize the connection between her symptoms and hormones—and do so a number of years before she expected to have to take midlife hormone changes into account. Many women are presently in this situation. And that's why I had to write this book.

PMS or Perimenopause?

"It's not unlike a bad case of premenstrual syndrome," said Gloria Bachman, professor and chief of obstetrics and gynecology at the Robert Wood Johnson Medical School in New Brunswick, New Jersey. Some of the most uncomfortable symptoms of a woman's midlife transition are present in its earliest stages, as noted by Gail Sheehy, author of the pioneering bestseller *The Silent Passage.* The suffering caused by the very real

Perimenopause Symptoms

Acne	Insomnia
Allergies	Irritability
Anger	Joint pain
Ankles or feet swollen	Leg cramps
Anxiety	Menstrual cycle irregularities
Backache	Migraines
Bloating	Memory problems
Blood sugar imbalance	Mood swings
Blood sugar level reduced	Muscular weakness
Bone loss	Night sweats
Breast sagging	Panic attacks
Breast tenderness	Sexual desire loss
Depression	Skin aging and dryness
Facial hair	Skin itching and crawling
Fatigue	Skin spots (liver or age spots)
Feelings of being crazy	Stomach cramps
Fibrocystic breast	Urinary incontinence
Fuzzy thinking	Urinary infections
Hair loss or thinning	Uterine fibroids
Headaches	Vaginal dryness
Heart palpitations	Water retention
Hot flashes	Weeping
Hypothyroidism	Weight gain
Hysteria	Weight loss inability

physical symptoms is made more intense by the bewilderment felt by women who have no idea that they have begun perimenopause. Sheehy said, "They feel—and in fact are—out of control of their bodies."

Indeed, many of the symptoms of perimenopause and premenstrual syndrome (PMS) are the same: bloating, weight gain, food cravings, headaches, depression, irritability, lack of energy, and loss of concentration. This is because both perimenopause and PMS are brought on by rising estrogen levels and a lack of progesterone. You can make a quick judgment about which is causing your symptoms with the following rule: If your periods continue to occur regularly, it's PMS. If your periods are irregular, it's perimenopause.

For *fully developed* perimenopause symptoms, remedying this lack of progesterone is usually the most direct and most effective form of therapy.

Although you can miss your period for a variety of reasons, including pregnancy, a continuing but irregular monthly cycle signals quite a different thing. Having such irregular periods is a strong reason to suspect that you have entered perimenopause. But entering perimenopause is not like entering a room. There's no door to open, and you are rarely conscious of crossing a threshold. Like many biological changes, this change is gradual—or, as some would say, insidious. Many women notice a pattern of "worsening PMS," starting as early as their midthirties, which is probably the beginning of ovarian hormonal shifts leading to perimenopause.

Quiz: Are You in Perimenopause?

Perimenopause should not be thought of as a disease or treated like one. It's a naturally occurring transition *before the change*. You can alleviate its symptoms in various ways, depending on how far along in the transition you are presently. Your answers to these questions will help you decide on your current status.

Scoring

Place the appropriate number in the Score column according to the intensity/frequency of your symptoms.

- Symptom is mild or occasional: 1

- Symptom is moderate or frequent: 2

- Symptom is severe: 3

Questions

After answering all ten questions, add up your total score.

Score

1. Do you feel depressed or have the "blues" for no apparent reason? _____

2. Do you experience restlessness, irritability, and anxiety? _____

3. Have your sleep patterns changed, with frequent awakenings or insomnia? _____

4. Does your heart sometimes pound while you are resting or sitting? _____

5. Do you have food cravings? _____

6. Do you have bloating or fluid retention? _____

7. Do you need to urinate more frequently? _____

8. Has your sex drive diminished? _____

9. Do you often have headaches or migraines? _____

10. Are you starting to put on weight around the middle? _____

Total Score _____

If you scored between 10 and 18: Don't worry, you're not going crazy. You are probably just beginning the perimenopause transition. A hormone-regulating diet and supplements, regular moderate exercise, and better management of stress may be all you need to alleviate your symptoms.

If you scored between 18 and 28: Diet, exercise, and stress management may or may not be enough to alleviate your symptoms. Additional nutrients and natural progesterone cream should make all the difference.

If you scored above 28: You are fully in perimenopause. The remedies above may be sufficient. If they are not, consider taking natural hormones. But first have a saliva test for hormone levels.

At What Age Will You Reach Menopause?

The Greek words *men pausis* mean "month to end," and *peri* means "near." Both perimenopause and menopause are stages in a longer process known as the climacteric. The climacteric refers to hormonal changes in a woman's body that take place from about age thirty-five to about age sixty. The average age of menopause for American women is fifty-one, but perimenopausal symptoms are felt by some women who are only thirty-five years old. There really is no way to tell at what age you will reach perimenopause.

Is there any way to tell at what age you will reach menopause? Your most likely age is your mother's age when she reached menopause. Heredity is important in this, but other factors are influential, too. Therefore, the more your health and lifestyle resemble those of your mother, the likelier it will be that heredity will be the deciding factor. Here are some factors that help cause menopause to come earlier. If many of these factors apply to your mother in her forties but not to you, you may reach menopause at a later age than she did. Unfortunately, the reverse also holds true. If more of these factors apply to you now than did to her in her forties, you may reach menopause earlier than she did.

Generally speaking, women who bear children after the age of forty and white women of northern European origin reach menopause at a later age than other American women. In some women, menopause can be abrupt. In others, at the opposite extreme, it can be a gradual transition spread over the years from about age thirty-five to age fifty. Both of these extremes are perfectly normal and healthy.

Individual perimenopausal differences among women do not reflect their comparative states of health. You can be extremely healthy and genetically or otherwise predisposed to perimenopausal symptoms. We need to keep in mind constantly that

Early Menopause Factors

	Your Mother	You
Smoke cigarettes		
Strict vegetarian		
Below normal cholesterol level		
Very thin athlete (especially marathon runner)		
Fashion-model thin		
Anorexic or bulimic		
Overweight		
Never had children		
Had late puberty		
African-American origin		
Mediterranean or southern European origin		
Lower socioeconomic background		
Pituitary gland problems		
Ovaries medically irradiated		

perimenopause is part of a natural process, not a pathological one.

More than 35 million women in America are presently in perimenopause. Despite this huge number, the medical community has only recently begun to recognize perimenopause as a distinct stage of a woman's life. Since many physicians are not aware of perimenopause as a stage of life, of course they do not recognize the symptoms that occur, such as moodiness, anxiety, weight gain, fuzzy thinking, and depression. Author and sex expert Lonnie Barbach says, "Perimenopause is an area of research that's totally infant. There's so little known."

Clinical and public interest in perimenopause has increased dramatically over the past five years. Since 1992, the Association of Reproductive Health Professionals (ARHP) has featured the latest research and medical information in its highly evaluated conference series, *Women's Health in the Perimenopause.*

You can also chalk up the change in attitude to the medical savvy and clout of the baby boomers, says Alan Altman, a Harvard Medical School gynecologist. Many of the women of this generation have recently entered the perimenopausal transition or will experience it soon. "Baby-boom women always demand answers," Altman told *McCall's* magazine. "Now they're asking, 'What's happening to my body and what can I do about it?' They want to take control of perimenopause, rather than allowing it to control them."

Which Hormones?

Once a woman has made the connection between her symptoms and hormones, it's easy for her to fall into a waiting trap. Instead of wondering exactly which hormones may be causing her symptoms, she may assume that sex hormones alone lie behind all her problems. She would probably be steered unconsciously to this assumption by all the magazine and television health pieces promoting hormone replacement therapy. Perhaps her doctor thinks it's a good idea. Physicians read all the time about the wonders of synthetic hormones, since much reading material is supplied to them by big pharmaceutical companies. But hormones other than sex hormones may be involved in her symptoms.

Which hormones? Any woman in her thirties or forties with symptoms for which a hormone imbalance is a likely cause needs to consider three different hormone systems. In the body, of course, these three hormone systems are all interconnected and influence one another in countless ways. We find it easier to think of them separately as follows:

Blood Sugar Hormones	**Adrenal Hormones**	**Ovarian Hormones**
Insulin	Stress hormones	Estrogen
Glucagon	Sex hormones	Progesterone
		Testosterone

Hormones are the chemical messengers of the body. They influence everything we think, feel, and do. In spite of that, we don't know much more about their intricate workings than we do about the surface of Mars. The more we learn about hormones, the more we find out how little we know.

We only have to look at the three hormone groups—blood sugar, adrenal, and ovarian—to see the obvious relationships among nutrition, stress, and sex hormones. (Both the adrenal glands and the ovaries secrete sex hormones.) One thing has constantly reminded me of this relationship, and that is the high level of complaints from women that hormone replacement therapy doesn't *feel right,* even after their symptoms have been alleviated. The only way I know for your body to feel right is to keep all therapeutic procedures as noninvasive and natural as possible. A balanced diet is the most healthful, cost-effective, and enjoyable form of therapy known. Most knowledgeable physicians would not be surprised to learn that what initially looked like a perimenopause symptom disappeared when the patient was placed on a balanced diet.

What I have observed many, many times is that women with imbalances of blood sugar or stress hormones have symptoms that are often indistinguishable from perimenopause symptoms. When these women eat a better diet or learn to manage their stress more effectively, they often are "miraculously" cured of their perimenopause symptoms.

In practical terms, it's a lot easier and much less expensive to balance your blood sugar hormones and stress hormones than your sex hormones.

Some Relevant Statistics About American Women

- There are more than 35 million perimenopausal women today.
- Eight out of ten perimenopausal women are sexually active.
- Nine out of ten perimenopausal women have had at least one child.
- More than one in four perimenopausal women are not married (one in seven women in their forties is divorced).
- Of *all* women aged 35 to 44: 29% smoke
  27% are overweight
  10% live in poverty

First, Do No Harm

As a professional nutritionist, I have devoted much of my time over the past twenty years to using nutritional therapy for female health problems. Twenty years ago, not many people—including women themselves—were willing to give priority to either female health problems or nutrition. Over those years, the slow-moving pendulum of medical opinion has swung almost completely in the other direction. But today many women still have health problems, and only a very small number are using the highly effective nutritional remedies available to them.

Although this book is mainly about how women can use nutritional therapy for perimenopause symptoms, I do not see nutrients as a cure for every condition. I do not take an inflexible stand, for instance, against hormone replacement therapy. I believe this kind of therapy should be used when a woman's health profile justifies it. When nutrition and exercise can give satisfactory relief from perimenopause symptoms, a woman ought not be put on a regimen of synthetic hormones. If a woman's body can heal itself in a natural way, an ancient philosophy of healing would argue against introducing something artificial into her body. "First, do no harm." That ancient instruction to healers holds true today.

A naturopathic doctor once remarked to me that using hormone replacement therapy for perimenopause symptoms that can be alleviated with nutrients and exercise is like using a crane to lift a teacup.

In This Book

In this book, we look first at how to get your blood sugar hormones in balance through eating a hormone-regulating diet. We see that no-fat and very-low-fat diets don't work because they are impossible to stay on for any length of time and often end in binges that leave the dieter worse off than before. An even greater problem created by no-fat and very-low-fat diets is that they deprive the body of good fats that it needs to manufacture hormones. In other words, too few good fats in your diet can contribute to your symptoms!

The diet world has been turned upside down by recognizing that the food we eat evokes a hormonal response inside our bodies. This seems a fairly obvious remark now, and we may need to be reminded that famous low-fat diets like those of Dean Ornish and Susan Powter (although helpful for some individuals with certain heart conditions) do not take the hormonal response to foods into account. We review the hormonal responses that nutrients evoke in our bodies—responses that make food the cheapest and most effective medicine available.

We next examine several essential nutrients that every woman must have in the correct amounts in order to feel emotionally and physically well. My professional experience has shown that these are the nutrients women are most likely to be deficient in. These nutrients help guarantee that a woman's diet is balanced and that her body has everything it needs to meet the challenges it faces. In my own nutritional practice, I often use tissue mineral analysis to reveal hidden imbalances in nutrient levels.

Moderate exercise helps all three hormone systems to function better. Indeed, exercise contributes positively to just about every bodily function and to most emotional and intellectual functions as well. Dr. Christiane Northrup claims that exercise for at least four hours a week lowers estrogen dominance (when skipped periods result in low progesterone levels). A high-fiber diet assists in this also. The secret of a good exercise program is to find something that you enjoy doing and that fits conveniently into your daily schedule. The more preparation that exercise requires, the easier it will be to find a reason to skip it today. But if you do something simple that you enjoy, you will *want* to do it every day. We show you how.

Stress levels are controlled by the adrenal hormones. The adrenals can become exhausted by overly stressful living, resulting in these glands not supplying sex hormones in the amounts needed, with consequent symptoms and additional stress building into a downward spiral. We show you how to rejuvenate your adrenal glands in two ways: through gland-renewing nutrients and by managing stressors in your life.

Eating a hormone-regulating diet, exercising moderately on a regular basis, and managing daily stress to some extent is often enough to alleviate the discomfort and symptoms felt by many women in their thirties and forties. However, diet, exercise, and stress management may not always be enough. When they are not enough, we show you how to resort to natural hormone therapy. Natural progesterone is usually the key therapeutic hormone, rather than estrogen. You can get natural progesterone creams over the counter without a prescription, and we list the most highly regarded brands for you. We also look at phytohormones (hormones from plants) and explain why they work.

In cases where not even natural progesterone cream and phytohormones are enough to alleviate the symptoms, women may need to take natural hormones directly, compounded specially for them on an individual basis. To discover what precisely her needs are, a woman needs to take hormone level tests. The new saliva test is best, and we show you why. We also show you how to take the test and how to find a pharmacist to make a hormonal remedy specially balanced for your needs.

Why not traditional hormone replacement therapy? We look at the risks involved, including that of breast cancer. We also acknowledge the reality that the vast majority of women stop taking prescription hormones within five years because they feel better without them.

The balance of the book is devoted to the Changing Diet Plan. The Changing Diet is the hormone-regulating diet that women need for their thirties and forties and beyond. The menus and recipes help you get started. The Changing Diet is loosely based on the 40/30/30 concept (40 percent carbohydrates, 30 percent fats, 30 percent protein), a food plan that is the focus of my recent booklet *The 40/30/30 Phenomenon* (New Canaan, CT: Keats, 1997). The Changing Diet is more oriented toward women's needs. This is not a one-diet-fits-all food plan. It can be adjusted for individual differences based upon ancestry, metabolic rate, and blood type. The diet is varied and fun—and requires very little time spent shopping and in the kitchen!

As you read on, you will find displayed ten tried and true remedies for perimenopausal symptoms. These ten remedies are displayed for your convenience because they are especially reliable, usually free of side effects, and easy to use. I call these remedies Peri Zappers. In the Roundup, we summarize the information on how Peri Zappers help balance the levels of three sets of hormones—blood sugar, stress, and ovarian—and how to use them to alleviate symptoms, look sleek and trim, and lead a more harmonious life.

Perimenopause can be a major challenge. But, as with any challenge, you can win and emerge from it looking physically great and feeling more emotionally fulfilled!

Chapter 2

Ann Louise's All-Star Peri Zappers

Perimenopausal symptoms are many, but the primary causes are relatively few. Only rarely do two women have exactly the same symptoms, while they may frequently share the same causes. But symptoms and their origins often cannot be tied together in a direct cause-and-effect relationship.

The fundamental cause of perimenopausal symptoms is hormonal imbalance, chiefly that between progesterone and estrogen in the menstrual cycle. The two most important causes of that hormonal imbalance are lack of regular ovulation and exhaustion of the adrenal glands.

Hormonal Imbalance

Estrogen and progesterone counter each other's effects. When their levels rise and fall as they should in a normal menstrual cycle, they are in balance and you do not suffer from symptoms. At most, you may have minor discomfort or inconvenience on menstruation. You don't have PMS or perimenopause symptoms at any time during the cycle.

An estrogen-progesterone balance gives you a symptom-free cycle, but it is, like all balances, subject to disruption when things go wrong. Eating a lot of processed carbohydrates and sugar causes an imbalance of estrogen and progesterone as well as of insulin. Poor eating habits, resulting in vitamin or mineral deficiencies, also cause an imbalance. So, too, do very-low-fat diets, which deprive the body of the good fats it needs to stay healthy and manufacture hormones. Stress can be a major problem, leaving its mark on the menstrual cycle. While women can go for years without showing any ill effects from an unhealthy lifestyle, poor nutrition, and high stress, the payoff is likely to be symptoms in their midthirties to late forties—the perimenopause years.

At some point during your perimenopause, you stop ovulating regularly. This can begin happening any time from your midthirties to your late forties. You may skip an occasional month or go two or more successive months without ovulating. When no egg ripens in your ovaries, there is no empty follicle to turn into a corpus luteum and secrete progesterone. This is when you start having mood swings, weight gain, and water retention.

Even when no ovulation occurs and no progesterone is secreted, the menstrual cycle proceeds. Estrogen causes the uterine lining to be shed, and menstrual flow takes place—though it may be very light or irregular. Then the brain sends a message to the ovaries, and a new cycle begins. You may go several cycles on estrogen alone. Author and physician John R. Lee called this situation estrogen dominance.

Some women have irregular periods for many years. They may notice light flow or only "spotting." Occasional heavy flows may signify ovulation and a return of progesterone. The fact that they are still menstruating causes many of these women to assume that their symptoms have nothing to do with hormones. Some women have few or no symptoms, while the lives of others are made miserable. And there are many grades between these two extremes.

When a woman doesn't ovulate for many successive months,

Dr. John R. Lee's List of Symptoms Caused or Made Worse by Estrogen Dominance

Aging process accelerated

Allergies

Autoimmune disorders (for example, lupus)

Blood clotting increase (raising risk of stroke)

Bone loss before menopause

Breast tenderness

Depression

Fat gain (especially around abdomen, hips, thighs)

Fatigue

Fibrocystic breasts

Foggy thinking

Gallbladder disease

Headaches

Hypoglycemia

Infertility

Irritability

Memory loss

Miscarriage

Osteoporosis

PMS

Sex drive decrease

Thyroid dysfunction mimicking hypothyroidism

Uterine cancer

Uterine fibroids

Water retention and bloating

---

her ovaries' secretion of estrogen can become erratic. She may have surges of the hormone, followed by unusually low levels. With estrogen surges, she is likely to suffer from water retention, weight gain, breast swelling and tenderness, sleep disturbance, and mood swings. But usually her estrogen levels remain normal, and the symptoms that she feels are caused mainly by her lack of progesterone.

If this woman has her hormone levels tested at a doctor's office, she will normally have lab tests ordered for the estrogen estradiol and for the follicle-stimulating hormone (FSH) and luteinizing hormone (LH), both brain messengers to the ovary. Only rarely will her progesterone level be measured. Depending on the stage of her cycle at which she is tested and on whether she is tested only once, which is usual, her estrogen level may appear low and her FSH high. In this event, the doctor may recommend that she take estrogen, which would be the last thing she needs in an already estrogen-dominant situation. Fortunately, the doctor is more likely to make a more benevolent misdiagnosis—that of emotional causes.

In remedying perimenopause symptoms, I take a holistic approach toward hormonal systems. By this, I mean that I don't approach symptoms as separate, independent entities, putting a patch on one here and another one there. Instead, I try to heal the underlying cause—by restoring the balance of three interconnected hormonal systems: ovarian, stress, and blood sugar hormones. I do this through the Changing Diet, which the second part of this book describes. Using the Changing Diet as an underlying stabilizing influence, I use a series of successive steps that I call Peri Zappers to cure perimenopause symptoms. I believe in starting out with the mildest remedy possible, that is, the Peri Zappers with low numbers.

The Peri Zappers are remedies based on my own personal experiences during perimenopause and on the experiences of thousands of women that I have assisted over the years as a nutritionist. As you read, you will meet the Zappers in numerical order, and you will see why they do the things they do. You will also meet a number of my clients, mentioned only by first name. All names, without exception, have been changed to protect the identities of the women involved. I take this opportunity to thank these women and many other clients who have shared with me so much by documenting their successful use of diet, nutrients, natural remedies, and exercise.

Liz

"I hate listening to people whine," Liz said, sitting across my desk from me. "I hate it even worse listening to myself do it."

"People don't come here to tell me about the wonderful things in their lives," I assured her.

She asked if she could smoke, and I said no. Liz gave me an appraising glance and said, "Look at my skin. Look how dry the skin on my arms is, and that's after I put on moisturizer only a couple of hours ago. Look at the wrinkles. Every day I see more of them. Look at my face. I'm forty-four. How old do I look to you?" She gazed at me with lackluster eyes. "I swear, every time I look in the mirror, I see myself *visibly* older than when I last looked at myself. It's like something out of a late-night horror movie."

"That's not necessarily aging, Liz," I said. "Your skin may be reflecting a deficiency in your body. Fix that deficiency, and your skin may recover."

"It's not just my skin," she went on. "My whole body is breaking down, falling to pieces. My mind, too. All at the same time! And I can't do anything about it!"

"I can—with your help," I volunteered.

"I hope so," she murmured, not sounding very convinced. "Let me tell you the rest, and maybe you won't be so sure. I've become fifteen pounds overweight in less than two years. That's fat. But if you'd seen me about ten days ago, I looked like I was thirty pounds overweight because of water retention. Then it went away. Also, I've been getting the most terrible headaches recently, right across the front of my forehead. And I get depressed. God, do I get depressed! It's not just feeling sorry for myself because I'm falling to pieces. This depression hits me from nowhere—drops on me like a black cloud and presses down on me!"

"I can help you," I said.

"There's one more thing," she warned. "I have no energy. I'm tired all the time. That's where I thought you could help, by giving me special vitamins and stuff that would at least get me up and going, so I could do something about all the other things, instead of sitting and staring into space."

"I can do better than that," I said. "Do you miss any periods?"

"Occasionally. Maybe twice a year."

We went on to talk about her lifestyle. Apart from cigarette smoking, frequent dieting was her main unhealthful pastime. When I told her that she didn't have a dozen different things wrong with her, but only one—unbalanced hormones—she probably didn't understand, and she certainly didn't believe me. But she agreed to follow my instructions, giving me six weeks to produce results. She would do everything I said except give up cigarettes.

I put her on the Changing Diet to help stabilize her hormones. Knowing that the diet on its own might not be sufficient in her case, I also had her include more of Peri Zapper #1, flaxseed oil. In only two weeks, she reported that her skin definitely looked smoother. Now, if only I could do something about her general well-being. . . . Although I usually recommend trying the Zappers in numerical order, I suggested that she skip to #5, natural progesterone cream, because this remedy is so all-encompassing and this woman wanted results yesterday. Nine or ten days later, she phoned to say that this was the magic potion she had been looking for. It was taking care of everything! Liz paid an office visit a month later. She looked like the younger sister of the woman I had seen previously. Even her hair had got back its sheen, and her eyes sparkled with life.

She was in such a tolerant mood, she even listened to what I had to say about smoking and promised to try a strategy I suggested. This involved switching to low-tar cigarettes and very gradually cutting back the number she smoked every day. If she could cut down to fifteen or fewer low-tars per day, she would no longer have a powerful nicotine addiction and would find it relatively easy to stop smoking by almost any method she chose.

More than a year later, Liz is still struggling with low-tars and occasional packs of not-so-lows, but she's getting there. She had much less struggle with her perimenopause symptoms, I'm glad to say. The Changing Diet, flaxseed oil, natural progesterone cream, and moderate exercise have made the symptoms more or less disappear. She also finds that B-complex vitamins seem to smooth over the rough surfaces.

My Background

Nutritionist Adele Davis was my first inspiration. From her I learned that food can heal, that stress is a big part of illness, and that you don't have to be sick or become helpless. Dr. Hazel Parcells, the respected "grand dame of alternative medicine," taught me the importance of parasites, heavy metals, and radiation as hidden causes of many ailments, including chronic fatigue, allergies, and blood sugar abnormalities. I also learned about the importance of the acid/alkaline balance at a cellular level.

Later in my career, as director of nutrition at the Pritikin Longevity Center in Santa Monica, I saw firsthand how diet and exercise can reverse serious conditions like cardiovascular disease, high blood pressure, and diabetes.

The late Nathan Pritikin, whose insight and benevolence remain an inspiration to me, was a pioneer of the low-fat diet. Dean Ornish is perhaps the best-known authority today on this kind of diet. The major drawback of the low-fat diet is that, if strictly adhered to, it is likely to shortchange your body of some essential fatty acids so vitally necessary for overall health. Besides, a very-low-fat diet is almost impossible to stay on for any length of time, because our bodily cravings overcome our mental resolutions. The problem then is that we are likely to binge on sugar-laden foods to compensate for the missing fats and eventually find ourselves worse off than we were before we started on the low-fat diet.

In my book *Beyond Pritikin,* I looked at the differences between "good" fats, which our bodies need, and "bad" fats, which cause health problems. That book, first published in 1988, emphasized the positive role of some fats in health and also raised early concern about the effects of eating so much grain, even the unprocessed, unrefined variety, on total health—a dietary approach that has evolved into the Changing Diet Plan that I introduce in this book. The Changing Diet Plan is a female version of the 40/30/30 diet (40 percent carbohydrates/30 percent fats/30 percent protein).

I set up my own practice after leaving the Pritikin Longevity Center. As well as seeing many clients, I reviewed the diet histories of more than seven thousand women in order to develop nutritional programs for various health problems, including weight gain, weight loss, eating disorders, irritable bowel syndrome, allergies, yeast infections, parasites, and premenstrual syndrome (PMS). My book *Super Nutrition for Women,* published in 1991, showed women how they could use nutrients to alleviate female symptoms that were still largely ignored by the medical profession at that late date.

While writing that book, I was struck by the comparatively large amount of nutritional research available for problems like PMS and yeast infections and the almost nonexistent supply of reliable nutritional information on menopause. Back in the mid–1960s, New York gynecologist Robert A. Wilson wrote a book entitled *Feminine Forever,* which popularized the notion that a menopausal woman without estrogen therapy became the female equivalent of a eunuch. The big pharmaceutical companies loved him.

By the early 1970s, many women were taking a combination of estrogen and tranquilizers as a remedy for premenstrual and menstrual symptoms. Then, in the mid–1970s, came the uterine cancer scare about estrogen and a decline in its use by women for several years. When research showed that taking synthetic progestin with estrogen protected women from uterine cancer, this form of therapy became increasingly widespread. Many women, however, found that they had been placed on a powerful, almost domineering, drug regimen, against which their bodies instinctively rebelled in subtle and not-so-subtle ways. From their bodies' reactions, these women learned that a less traumatic, less invasive, more natural cure was needed. Today this natural cure is possible, since much more is known about human, animal, and plant hormones.

That was certainly not the case in 1992, when I had reached the big forty and was writing *Super Nutrition for Menopause*. I used the relatively small amount of nutritional research published at that time and relied on my own experience with clients and that of other medical researchers to suggest milder, more natural, less invasive remedies for menopausal symptoms.

I have maintained a private practice for more than twenty years on both the West coast and the East Coast. Much of my work in recent years has centered around custom-tailoring diets to fit your body's special needs. My book *Your Body Knows Best* is an individualized approach to weight loss. This involves taking your metabolic rate, blood type, and ancestry into account when assessing which diet is right for your body.

Meet the Peri Zappers

You already know that you'll be meeting the Peri Zappers in numerical order as you read through the text. But here's a short introduction to each of the members of this all-star team. There are no rookies here! All these Zappers are combat-hardened veterans from the symptom wars. Don't forget that they work best when you are on the Changing Diet—which appears in the second part of this book.

Peri Zapper #1:
Flaxseed Oil

The healing oil of flaxseed contains both omega–3 and –6 fatty acids and is the chemical precursor of the fatty acid EPA and of hormonelike prostaglandins. Flaxseed oil is a great remedy for perimenopausal symptoms, especially skin conditions, depression, and fatigue. But it also fights cancer, lowers cholesterol levels, makes insulin more effective, and boosts the immune system. You can use flaxseed oil as a salad dressing or as a topping for veggies and grains and in no-heat recipes.

Peri Zapper #2:
Evening Primrose Oil

Some of my clients swear by this healing oil. It contains the fatty acid GLA, which converts into hormonelike prostaglandins. I believe that GLA is a miracle ingredient, especially for cramping, irritability, headaches, and water retention. It is most potent in its preformed state in evening primrose oil, although the raw material for GLA can be found in some unprocessed vegetable oils.

Peri Zapper #3:
M 'n' M (Multivitamins and Magnesium)

A combo of certain vitamins and magnesium may be necessary to get your hormonal systems back in balance. M 'n' M is a marvelous tonic for the mind as well as the body, helping to smooth out mood swings, insomnia, anxiety, tissue dryness, and water retention.

Vitamin B complex, including 50 to 100 milligrams of vitamin B_6

Vitamin C, 1000 milligrams three times a day

Vitamin E, 400 to 1200 international units

Magnesium, 500 to 1000 milligrams before sleeping

Peri Zapper #4:
Think Zinc

If M 'n' M doesn't completely clear up your symptoms, you should try a zinc supplement. This mineral is a must if you are vegetarian, because your diet is often lacking in it. Zinc (15 to 50 milligrams a day) helps to lower estrogen and increase progesterone levels, build strong bones, and keep your immune system in tiptop shape to ward off viruses.

Peri Zapper #5:
Natural Progesterone Cream

In perimenopause, your symptoms are frequently due to a low progesterone level. Taking an artificial progesterone (progestin) can intensify your symptoms and also make your body feel that something is not quite right. Natural progesterone is the same molecule as that in our bodies. Taken as a nonprescription skin cream, it rebuilds your body's progesterone level, restores hormonal balance, and helps relieve a wide array of symptoms, including decreased sex drive, depression, abnormal blood sugar levels, fatigue, fuzzy thinking, irritability, thyroid dysfunction, water retention, bone loss, fat gain, and low adrenal function.

Peri Zapper #6:
Exercise

Be vigorously active for a half hour, five days a week. Do housework, garden, walk briskly, cycle, swim, dance, have fun. Do different things each day—and do what you enjoy!

Peri Zapper #7:
Destressing Stress

Take a good look and see if you can interrupt the three-step stressor-distress-consequence process.

Peri Zapper #8:
Adrenal Refresher

When you are under a lot of stress, replacing lost minerals and vitamins can help your adrenal glands secrete stress hormones.

Peri Zapper #9:
Soy Phytoestrogens

Soybeans and certain other plants are rich in mild plant estrogen, which can occupy your cell estrogen receptors and reduce the undesirable effects of estrogen. Natural progesterone can also counteract estrogen. Additionally, phytohormones can help balance fluctuating hormone levels.

Peri Zapper #10:
Natural Hormone Therapy

You still don't have to take horse estrogen and artificial progesterone (progestin), subjecting yourself to a risk of breast cancer and to weird bodily feelings. You can take natural hormones, specially prepared for your needs as indicated by saliva tests of your hormone levels.

Finding Zappers

When you need to find a Peri Zapper in a hurry, say, to check the specific dosage of something, you'll find them listed in succession in the Roundup section at the back of the book. If you need to check on something in the discussion about a particular Zapper, riffle through the pages while looking for the distinctive design, with all those stars.

Although the Zappers are presented in ascending order of strength, don't automatically assume that the strongest is the one you must try because of your severe symptoms. Time and time again, I have found the mildest Zappers work miracles, especially when taken in conjunction with the changing diet—a powerful hormone balancer in and of itself.

Chapter 3

Curbing Carbs

*The Forty Percent Solution
for Weight Gain, Munchies,
and Short Attention Span*

Surprisingly, symptoms like depression, mood swings, and even weight gain may have just as much to do with your diet as with perimenopause itself. These symptoms often seem to go away by themselves when you switch to a blood sugar or hormone-balancing eating plan. So many clinical research studies have associated both depression and mood swings with hypoglycemia, or low blood sugar, that I would be remiss if I did not present diet as a mainline therapy. Avoiding low blood sugar is critical, because sugar (glucose) is the body's main fuel source. When blood sugar levels start to drop, the brain becomes frantic for its only source of fuel—and that's when sugar cravings and bingeing begin. Ironically, some of those highly touted complex carbohydrates can create the same blood sugar peaks and valleys as sweets, because of their glycemic response (more about this later) and the insulin connection.

During the low blood sugar period, you can feel mood swings, irritability, and lack of attention and even undergo a weight shift. This roller-coaster ride of high and low blood sugar is caused by hormones reacting to the food you have eaten—primarily reactions between carbohydrates and the pancreatic hormone insulin, between proteins and the pancreatic hormone glucagon, and between fats and the hormones called eicosanoids. (All of this will be covered in this chapter and the next.) A fundamental solution to your symptoms, whether they are related to blood sugar or perimenopause, is an eating plan that consists of slow-acting or low-glycemic carbohydrates, along with high-quality fats and proteins that keep insulin levels low and that help to stabilize blood sugar levels.

For the past twenty years, most women in the perimenopause stage—from the late thirties to the late forties—have been brainwashed about the benefits of a low-fat, high-complex-carbohydrate diet plan. I believe that this is precisely the very unbalanced eating regimen that has created many of the symptoms that we are now attributing to perimenopause.

With the help of the media and even some federal agencies, the words *low fat* have became almost synonymous with *healthful diet* in America. When people hear mention of dietary fats, they immediately think of cholesterol, heart disease, or obesity. Significant numbers of people have set about changing their eating habits by cutting fat from their diets. Many develop food cravings, and some go on eating binges. Those who stay on the low-fat diet make up for the missing fats by devouring large amounts of carbohydrates, such as bread, muffins, bagels, fat-free cookies, and low-fat yogurt.

Even today, large numbers of otherwise careful eaters think it's just fine to load up on fat-free but high-glycemic carbohydrates, such as rice cakes, corn, and whole-grain bread. They don't realize that many of the complex carbohydrates they eat act in the same way as processed simple carbohydrates by causing a surge in their blood sugar levels. Their elevated blood sugar levels are answered by a rise in blood insulin levels. The hormone insulin stops the body from burning stored body fat as fuel, causing a sharp drop in blood sugar level. This causes the brain to signal for more blood sugar to use as an easy fuel, which they feel as a craving for something sweet. And this is when they reach for a high-sugar snack or soft drink.

When I was director of nutrition at the Pritikin Longevity Center in Santa Monica in the early 1980s, I first noticed that many people on a diet low in fat and high in complex carbohydrates often suffered from low energy, fatigue, mood swings, allergies, yeast infections, and dry skin, hair, and nails. I wrote about them in my first book, *Beyond Pritikin,* and I believe that their symptoms were caused by a lack of essential fatty acids that we normally get in the "good" dietary fats and an overemphasis on carbohydrates from such allergenic grains as wheat and from fermented seasonings.

These individuals may be regarded as extreme examples, of course, because the early Pritikin diet was so severe, since it was originally designed to be therapeutic. In general, however, it remains true that the health of Americans has not improved in proportion to the increasing popularity of low-fat diets. In fact, the opposite is true. Best-selling author and physician Robert C. Atkins, among others, has pointed out that Americans are more obese now than ever before (one in three, up from one in four a decade ago), diabetes has tripled in the past thirty years, more people are getting cancer, heart disease rates are unchanged, and low-grade ailments like chronic fatigue syndrome and food sensitivities are on the rise. I would add attention deficit hyperactivity disorder (ADHD) to this woeful list. An excess of carbohydrates and sugar, affecting the body's insulin response, may be a major contributory cause of ADHD. I would also mention the increasing incidence of parasites. Many worms and microscopic organisms thrive in a sugar-rich environment, and Americans presently eat 150 pounds of sugar per person per year.

Diane

An accountant for a chain of stores, Diane put in many sedentary hours at her work. But she made up for it in her free time, she told me. At forty-one, she walked briskly a few miles with her husband every day, rain or shine, year round. I could see that she needed to lose at least fifteen pounds. She had broad shoulders, a low waistline, and short legs—the kind of body that would look almost square if she put on much more weight. Diane's manner was at first outgoing and attractive, but then she seemed to lapse into a sort of tiredness, even despondency, after only a few minutes of conversation with me.

"I can't lose weight, no matter what I try," she told me. "Every time I relax my vigilance with food, I put on another pound, which of course I then can't lose. So I went to a dietitian. She put me on a low-fat diet and had me getting 55 percent of my calories from carbs, 20 percent from protein, and 25 percent from fats. You know what happened? I began to feel tired all the time. So I quit the dietitian."

"And then what happened?" I prompted her.

She sighed. "I tried other low-fat diets, but by now I was beginning to be peppered by moody fits and lack of concentration. To tell you the truth, I began to wonder if I wasn't suffering from adult attention deficit disorder, especially after I read about it in a magazine. This has been going on now for more than a year, and I can feel that I'm getting worse. I started out being worried about my weight. Weight is the least of my worries now. I'm an accountant, and I can't concentrate!"

I sympathized with her, having had numerous clients with similar experiences. When I asked what she ate on a typical workday, she gave me the following portrait of her eating habits.

> *Breakfast*: A cup of coffee with skim milk and corn flakes with a sliced banana.
> *Midmorning*: To combat tiredness, a fat-free bran muffin.
> *Lunch*: Salad (no dressing, of course), pasta with meatless marinara, and broccoli with no butter or oil.
> *Midafternoon*: A low-fat yogurt as a pick-me-up.
> *Dinner*: Lots of veggies stir-fried in a Teflon pan, with lots of brown rice and one ounce of skinless chicken.
> *After dinner*: Famished, she made frequent trips to the refrigerator for fat-free ice cream, cookies, and so forth.

I pointed out to her that basically all she was eating was sugar, sugar, sugar. Even the complex carbs—for example, brown rice at dinner—were fast acting or high-glycemic. I finally talked her into an egg for breakfast or some natural peanut butter on an apple wedge as she was flying out the door. For lunch, she needed chicken, tuna, or seafood. At midafternoon, some almonds. For a normal dinner, I suggested salad, lean veal, green vegetables, and a small sweet potato. I pleaded with her to put a teaspoon of olive oil on her salads and to eat nuts.

"Watch your carb portions," I warned her.

In eyeballing her portions, she needed to recognize that an average-size portion of chicken, beef, or fish was about the size of a deck of cards. A serving of vegetables and starchy food, such as pasta, potatoes, or corn, should be no bigger than a tennis ball. In this serving, ideally there should be three times as much vegetables as starchy food. A teaspoon of oil is about the size of a quarter.

With a little practice, such visual estimates of plate content become easy and almost second nature. They are of great value in eating out, when you can ease excess quantities to one side of your plate and avoid overeating or unbalanced eating. A food that is fat free, like pasta or rice, needs to be portion controlled because the insulin response can prompt the body to store excess calories as body fat.

In less than a week, Diane had made a total diet transition. That was all the time it took on her new diet to break the habit of nighttime refrigerator visits. In less than a month, she noticed the difference in her powers of concentration at work. She thought that she had lost about a pound. In another couple of weeks, Diane was sure. She was losing weight!

Diane continued to do well. When I last saw her, about a year ago, she was bubbly and bright, as well as trim and active. It had been a long time since she had last felt tired, moody, or depressed.

Carbohydrates and Blood Sugar

All carbohydrates are converted by the body into blood sugar in the form of glucose. In a balanced state, our bloodstream contains about two teaspoons of glucose. The carbohydrates that we eat easily supply this amount of glucose and all too easily exceed the amount we need. The blood sugar glucose that our body does not use as fuel is stored as body fat, under the control of the hormone insulin. With our bodies' blood sugar requirements so easily met, the last thing we need to eat is simple sugars, processed carbohydrates (white flour, pasta, white rice), or excessive amounts of potatoes, corn chips, or brown rice. All these carbohydrates rapidly convert into glucose and cause a sharp rise in our blood sugar level, followed by a sharp rise in our insulin level, followed in turn by storage of excess blood sugar as body fat. This is why people who eat a lot of low-fat pasta dishes can actually put on weight instead of losing it!

At this point, some people throw up their hands in despair. What are they to do? The first step is simply to accept two facts: (1) there are good and bad dietary fats, and our bodies need the good ones; and (2) the food we eat evokes a hormonal response in our bodies. The next step is to move away from a low-fat diet of 55 percent carbohydrates, 20 percent protein, and 25 percent (or less) fats toward a hormone-regulating diet of 40 percent carbohydrates, 30 percent protein, and 30 percent fats. These percentages are approximate proportions for the three macronutrients and should not be interpreted as strict mathematical quantities.

Telling good fats from bad is easy, as we will see in the next chapter. It's less easy to get familiar with the different types of carbohydrate foods. Which of them evoke rapid blood sugar and insulin responses, and which are digested more slowly and therefore evoke a less steep rise in blood sugar and, consequently, a less steep rise in the fat storage hormone insulin? The glycemic index is the best way to get to know this aspect of carbohydrates.

Glycemic Index

Of the three basic kinds of nutrients—carbohydrates, proteins, and fats—carbohydrates are by far the richest source of blood sugar. Carbohydrates are of two kinds, simple and complex. Simple carbohydrates (often termed simple sugars) are built of one or two molecules. They are digested and absorbed by the body quickly, providing a rush of blood sugar. Complex carbohydrates consist of chains of simple sugars. They vary in the speed with which they are digested and absorbed by the body. In the glycemic index, carbohydrate foods are classified into three main groups according to the rapidity with which they are turned into blood sugar by the body. The higher a food appears on the index, the faster it induces insulin and therefore the greater its undesirability as a food.

You will probably need to look at the glycemic index a few times before it begins to make good sense to you. As you become more familiar with the index, you will be able to assign a place on it for foods not listed. Getting to understand the overall picture is much more important than remembering whether one food is several steps up or down from another. The glycemic index is an instant reference telling you which foods to eat plentifully, moderately, or as little as possible. The index even permits you to cheat by combining a desirable high-glycemic food with low-glycemic foods so that the total stays within bounds. More important, it can save you from unknowingly eating several high-glycemic foods together in one meal. The glycemic index here is adapted from my book *Beyond Pritikin*.

The Glycemic Index of Foods

RAPID INDUCERS OF INSULIN

Glycemic index greater than 100 percent

Puffed rice	40% bran flakes
Corn flakes	Rice Krispies
Maltose	Weetabix
Puffed wheat	Tofu ice cream substitute
French baguette	Millet
Instant white rice	

Glycemic index of 100 percent

Glucose	Whole-wheat bread
White bread	

Glycemic index between 90 and 99 percent

Grape-Nuts
Carrots
Parsnips
Barley (whole-meal)

Muesli
Shredded wheat
Apricots
Corn chips

Glycemic index between 80 and 89 percent

Rolled oats
Oat bran
Honey
White rice
Brown rice
White potato

Corn
Rye (whole-meal)
Shortbread
Ripe banana
Ripe mango
Ripe papaya

Glycemic index between 70 and 79 percent

All-Bran
Kidney beans
Wheat (coarse)

Buckwheat
Oatmeal cookies

MODERATE INDUCERS OF INSULIN

Glycemic index between 60 and 69 percent

Raisins
Mars candy bars
Spaghetti (white)
Spaghetti (whole-wheat)
Pinto beans
Macaroni
Rye (pumpernickel)

Bulgur
Couscous
Wheat kernels
Beets
Apple juice
Applesauce

Glycemic index between 50 and 59 percent

Potato chips
Barley
Green banana
Lactose
Peas (frozen)

Sucrose
Yam
Custard
Dried white beans

Glycemic index between 40 and 49 percent

Sweet potato   Oatmeal (steel-cut)
Navy beans   Sponge cake
Peas (dried)   Butter beans
Bran   Grapes
Lima beans   Oranges
Rye (whole-grain)   Orange juice

REDUCED INSULIN SECRETION

Glycemic index between 30 and 39 percent

Apples   Chickpeas
Pears   Milk (skim)
Tomato soup   Milk (whole)
Ice cream   Yogurt
Black-eyed peas   Fish sticks (breaded)

Glycemic index between 20 and 29 percent

Lentils   Peaches
Fructose   Grapefruit
Plums   Cherries

Glycemic index between 10 and 19 percent

Soybeans   Peanuts

People are often startled by some of the food rankings when they first look at the glycemic index. For example, they may be surprised to find that brown rice is higher on the scale than a Mars bar! This ranking simply means that brown rice evokes a more rapid insulin response than a Mars bar. The candy bar contains fats (mostly bad) that slow down the insulin response. The glycemic index does not take into account whether these fats are good or bad, only that they slow down the insulin response. Therefore we need to keep in mind that the glycemic index is not an overall seal of approval of foods, but strictly a ranking of foods according to their ability to evoke an insulin response in the bloodstream.

When you consult the glycemic index, you may find the following key points worth keeping in mind.

o Proteins and fats eaten with high- or moderate-glycemic foods help slow down the body's absorption of carbohydrates. This in turn discourages sharp rises in blood sugar and insulin levels.

o The kind of energy you feel has a lot to do with the glycemic index of the foods you eat. High-glycemic foods deliver a faster burst of energy and a quicker letdown. The lower on the glycemic index a food is placed, the more it provides a healthier, more long-term kind of energy.

Insulin Resistance and Other Disorders

Simple sugars, processed carbohydrates, and high-glycemic carbohydrates, when eaten alone, cause a flood of glucose to be released into the bloodstream. The pancreas responds to this blood sugar imbalance by secreting the hormone insulin. The hormone restores the blood sugar balance by helping to send the glucose in two directions: to muscles to be consumed as fuel for energy and to adipose tissue to be stored as body fat.

The human insulin system evolved over thousands of years to process nutrients from natural, unprocessed foods, which it does very efficiently. But insulin has not yet had time to adapt to nutrients from modern foods, particularly the large amount of carbohydrates from grains. Until humans became agrarian, which took place comparatively late in our development, carbohydrates from grains were only a small part of our diet.

Frequent alternation of blood sugar/insulin highs and lows from eating too many simple sugars and processed and high-glycemic carbohydrates is thought to cause insulin resistance after a while. The body becomes progressively less sensitive to insulin, and increasing amounts of the hormone are required to process the glucose. Insulin resistance is believed to be responsible when, as in many cases, overweight people cannot lose weight on a low-fat, high-carbohydrate diet. Some experts estimate that as many as one in four Americans have insulin resistance to some extent, while a few high estimates place the rate at three in four.

Adult-onset diabetes is another problem associated with diet and blood sugar. Sixteen million Americans are thought to have the disorder, only half of whom know it. The National Center for Health Statistics says that 59,000 Americans died of diabetes in 1995. In a six-year Harvard study that tracked the diets of 65,173 women aged forty to sixty-five, Dr. Jorge Salmeron and co-workers found that women who ate a starchy diet low in fiber and who drank a lot of soda developed diabetes two and a half times more often than similar women who ate a more healthful diet.

Obesity is strongly linked to adult-onset diabetes, which affects twice as many women as men over the age of forty-five. In cases of obesity, weight loss alone can be enough to control or cure the condition. Perimenopause is certainly the time when a woman needs to check whether her diet regulates her blood sugar hormones. Getting these hormones in balance now with the Changing Diet does much to ensure good health in future years.

If you think that you might be diabetic or a borderline case, visit your doctor for a blood test of your blood sugar levels while fasting. A second test while fasting at a different time on another day is good for a comparison measurement. A glucose level greater than 130 milligrams per 100 milliliters of blood indicates a diabetic condition. A glucose level of 100 to 130 milligrams per 100 milliliters of blood indicates a borderline diabetic condition.

Hypoglycemia, cardiovascular disease, and impaired immunity are other conditions linked to diet and blood sugar. Women often eat too much fruit because they think that since fruit is natural, large amounts must be all the better for you. However, too much fruit can upset the body's delicate calcium balance and raise blood triglyceride levels. High triglyceride levels in women caused by excessive carbohydrates are a major risk factor for heart disease, which becomes the number one killer of women later in life.

Too much fruit also encourages the growth of yeast. If you have a yeast problem, avoid all fruit for at least ten days or eat no more than one fruit a day.

As we gain increasing knowledge of hormones, we are likely to get a better understanding of the symptoms that many disorders share with perimenopause. In the meantime, it is enough to know that diet, hormones, and the presence or absence of many female symptoms are all interconnected. It may be many years before researchers have worked out all the intricate and marvelous interactions of blood sugar, stress, and ovarian hormones—and how these interactions differ from woman to woman. I'm convinced that one day we will know all this. My strategy in the Changing Diet has been to take as broad an approach as possible to regulating hormones through nutrition and to dismiss few possibilities, not holding back to quibble over fine points that may be regarded as irrelevant in a year.

Fiber

Fiber, or "roughage," as my grandmother used to say, is not simply indigestible hulks and skins. Fiber comes in several different kinds, and our bodies need them all to stay in good health. Cellulose is the indigestible kind of fiber in nearly all vegetables and fruit; this is usually what we mean when we say *fiber*. But we shouldn't ignore the other kinds of fiber that the human digestive system can partially break down. Found mixed with cellulose in various foods, they include lignins, pectins, gums, and hemicelluloses.

Dietary fiber is known to lower estrogen dominance, a condition suffered by many women during perimenopause. Fiber binds to excess estrogens and helps to eliminate them from the body. Additionally, David P. Rose of the American Health Foundation in New York found that two months on a high-fiber diet reduced levels of the less desirable form of estrogen estrone without affecting the levels of either progesterone or the more desirable form of estrogen estriol.

In recent years fiber has been acknowledged as a potent fighter of cancer by helping to remove potentially dangerous substances from the intestines. Even more recently, this poor relation of carbohydrates has been in the limelight as a regulator of blood sugar hormones.

The director of the Harvard study mentioned above, Dr. Walter Willett, a professor of epidemiology and nutrition at the

Harvard School of Public Health, told the *New York Times* that fiber also slowed the absorption of carbohydrates and prevented surges in the levels of blood sugar and insulin. He added that micronutrients in fiber, particularly magnesium, may help prevent diabetes. Other studies have shown that magnesium makes the body more sensitive to insulin, which lessens the need for the pancreas to secrete more of the hormone. Dr. Willett suggested that magnesium gained from fiber was probably more beneficial than that from supplements.

As we have seen, the kinds and amounts of carbohydrates that we eat are of prime importance in a hormone-regulating diet. Desirable high-fiber foods on the Changing Diet include moderate and low-glycemic complex carbohydrates such as chick-peas, pinto beans, lentils, rye, whole-grain spaghetti, barley, yams, fruits, and vegetables.

Chapter 4

Hormone-Friendly Proteins and Fats

Improving Sleep, Memory, Skin Tone, and Hair Tone

oth carbohydrates and fats play major roles in the body's generation of energy. Although proteins can be consumed as fuel for energy, this is neither effective nor desirable. The functions of proteins in human body chemistry are very different from those of carbohydrates and fats, yet their relationship to hormones is even closer.

If your body does not get enough protein from the food you eat, its ability to make new proteins slows down and it may even break down existing body protein (such as muscle tissue) to supply its needs. If your body starts breaking down its own muscle tissue, your metabolism slows down further, with the result that you burn fewer calories and fat. This is how a diet too high in carbohy-drates and low in proteins can cause a loss of muscle tone. Other symptoms resulting from too little protein in the diet include thinning skin, brittle nails, loss of hair, food cravings, loss of sex-ual desire, fatigue, irritability, and mental confusion.

You need to eat part of your daily total requirement of protein at each meal. If you skip your breakfast or lunch protein, intend-ing to make up for it at dinner, your body will store fat instead of using it as fuel.

Alice

For about six months, Alice had been losing her hair. At first, the loss had been hardly noticeable—a few extra hairs to be pulled from a comb or brush. Within a couple of months, there were a lot more hairs to be pulled from her comb and brush, plus more caught in the drain after she took a shower. At forty-three, Alice was proud of her shoulder-length jet black hair, without a single strand of gray, which she wore in a ponytail when active but pre-ferred to wear loose. But now the least bit of pressure pulled it out by the roots! Her husband said it was probably stress from her new job as assistant principal at the local junior high school. Alice felt that, if anything, she encountered less stress in this new posi-tion than she had as a regular classroom teacher.

Then Alice began to notice that the muscles of her thighs and upper arms were becoming less firm than they had been. Her hus-band asked if her new job was more sedentary than classroom work. It seemed to her that she was never off her feet, rushing from one part of the school to another to resolve an unending stream of minor problems. She was sure it wasn't lack of exercise that was causing her muscles to become flabby.

Her family doctor could find no medical cause for her hair loss or flabby muscles. On the chance that these symptoms might have something to do with an early beginning of menopause, he recom-mended that she see her gynecologist. Noting that her menstrual cycle was more or less regular, her gynecologist dismissed this pos-sibility. She told Alice to come back the following week when the results of her lab tests would be available. All the results came back normal. At a loss, the gynecologist suggested that she see a nutritionist.

A friend of Alice's had been a client of mine and referred her to me. Determined to find relief, Alice drove more than two hundred miles to see me.

When I asked Alice about her daily diet, I began to see why her gynecologist had recommended a nutritionist. Alice ate what amounted to a vegan diet, with beans and other legumes as her only source of protein. If she had been healthy on such a diet, I would have had little to say. But she was not healthy and, as I soon found out, did not associate any of her symptoms with her meager diet. In fact, the opposite was true. She was convinced that were it not for her strict vegetarianism, her symptoms would be worse.

Alice didn't have any ethical reasons not to eat animal products. Having heard that vegetarian women have the strongest bones, she had gone on a vegetarian diet as an anti-aging strategy. I explained that her diet was probably largely responsible for her hair loss and flabby muscles. Alice had a fast metabolism and type B blood, and that could explain why vegetarianism had not worked for her. (Chapter 15 discusses how individual differences, including differences in metabolism and blood type, influence a person's bodily responses to food.) I suggested that she should eat small amounts of protein at every meal, such as fish, eggs, or organic turkey. As a safety measure, because of her age, I also suggested that she try natural progesterone cream (discussed in Chapter 7). In less than two weeks, her hair loss began to ease and her thigh and upper-arm muscles regained some firmness. In six to seven weeks, she was back to normal. Since that time—four years ago—Alice has maintained her health with a protein-rich diet. She remarked to me that she no longer had a tendency to put on weight, although she had never complained of this as a symptom. (Women so often don't describe *all* their symptoms!) I said that it was probably due to protein stimulating the hormone glucagon to mobilize body fat to be burned as fuel.

Alice's gynecologist was unusual in that she suggested to a patient that she see a nutritionist, although physicians increasingly recognize nutrition as a complementary therapy if a patient suggests it. But I found it encouraging that the gynecologist recommended a nutritionist to review her eating habits. Good sign!

Proteins

Hormones and other hormonelike chemical messengers in the body, such as neurotransmitters and prostaglandins, actually are proteins. Human proteins are made up of twenty-two different kinds of amino acids, eight of which the body cannot make itself and must obtain from food. These eight are thus called essential amino acids. While the body absorbs proteins whole from both animal and plant food, it does not use them whole. Instead, it breaks them down into amino acids and reassembles its own proteins from these. Amino acids are also widely used by the body without being resynthesized as proteins.

The Eight Essential Amino Acids That Make Up Proteins

Isoleucine	Phenylalanine
Leucine	Threonine
Lysine	Tryptophan
Methionine	Valine

Since our bodies don't store amino acids as they do carbohydrates and fat, we need to get a constant supply of these eight essential amino acids in our food. This is another good reason to make sure you get some high-quality protein with every meal.

The amino acids that make up protein are called the "building blocks of life" because the body uses them to rebuild and repair its tissues and organs. If water were removed from a human body, more than half of its dry weight would be protein. Our skin, hair, nails, muscles, hormones, metabolic enzymes, and neurotransmitters are all composed of some of the more than fifty thousand proteins that the body makes use of.

Proteins perform many life-giving functions inside our bodies. Because of what we have learned about carbohydrates and blood sugar, it's worth pointing out that proteins, like fats, have a stabilizing effect on blood sugar, producing steady, long-term energy instead of a short burst and a quick letdown.

Proteins also stimulate the secretion by the pancreas of the hormone glucagon, which works in opposition to insulin. What insulin stores in body fat, glucagon puts back into the bloodstream for use as fuel. Glucagon releases the fat-stored sugar glycogen into the bloodstream to restore the blood sugar level, and also releases fat from adipose tissue. This fat, burned as fuel, then disappears.

It's interesting to compare the functions of insulin and glucagon:

Functions of Insulin and Glucagon

Insulin	Glucagon
Lowers blood sugar level	Raises blood sugar level
Stores fat	Mobilizes fat from storage
Triggered by carbohydrates	Triggered by proteins

Adult protein requirements tend to be much underestimated in traditional low-fat diets. Approximately 30 percent of calories should be derived from proteins in a hormone-regulating diet. Proteins provide four calories per gram. In the Changing Diet, you will be delighted by protein in the form of low-fat cottage and ricotta cheeses, lean red meat, poultry, seafood, fish, soy, whey, and eggs.

Jessica

A client called to say that a close friend would be contacting me for an appointment. Hardly five minutes later, the phone rang. Jessica sounded overwrought and begged to see me immediately on an emergency basis. I gently raised the possibility of her visiting a hospital emergency clinic, but she told me it wasn't "that kind" of emergency. I agreed to add her at the end of an already overcrowded day's schedule.

When Jessica walked into my office, she looked so miserable I was glad I worked her in because I felt I could help her. She was fashionably thin and wore a loose silk designer dress and expensive Italian shoes, but her hair looked dull and lifeless and her skin was dry and wrinkled. She looked like she was in her early fifties. Her beautiful clothes just made things worse by creating a contrast. She told me she was thirty-eight. I'd seen women aged fifty-five with better skin and hair.

"My mother came to stay with us for a few days," she told me. "We hadn't seen her for a couple of years. She has a sharp tongue, and my husband and two kids kept out of her way as much as they could. I wish I could have, too. She was hardly in the house an hour before I became the target. She said I'd aged ten years since she saw me last."

I nodded encouragingly. But, so far, her mother sounded to me like a reasonably observant person.

"Anyway, she kept harping on and on about my appearance and premature aging," Jessica continued, becoming visibly more upset as she recalled events. "I could hardly wait to drive her to the airport yesterday morning. We got there nearly three hours before her plane was due to take off, and I just left her there without waiting with her."

"Did your husband hear what she said about you?" I asked.

"I was coming to that," she said. "In a roundabout, diplomatic kind of way, obviously trying to spare my feelings, he said to me that I should listen to what my mother had said. Well, then I flipped out, screaming that it was for him I was trying to be elegant and beautiful—so that he could be proud to be seen with me!"

Jessica had nice eyes, a narrow face, and long fingers. With her expensive clothes, she would have been very chic and elegant anywhere, if it weren't for the condition of her skin and hair, which aged her beyond her years.

She mentioned her friend's name. "She started with me at the diet clinic but dropped out after only a couple of weeks," Jessica said. "She told me that was when she started coming to see you. I had coffee with her this morning and told her about the things my mother had been saying, and that was when she compared her neck and hands to mine. She didn't have to say anything else. I asked for your phone number."

"That was the emergency?"

"You bet." She gave me a small smile. "Can you help?"

I was familiar with the very-low-fat diet that Jessica was rigorously following. It was a fashionable one, often mentioned in glossy magazines in association with supermodels and Hollywood stars. Its appeal to Jessica was not hard to figure. Some of its adherents, including Jessica apparently, regarded all fat in food as more or less toxic. As a result of this overzealousness, their bodies had lower than healthy levels of certain fatty acids that the body does not make itself. These so-called essential fatty acids are necessary for the body's manufacture of important molecules that are the building blocks of hormones and other substances. In trying to avoid all fats, Jessica had probably deprived herself of even the good ones.

But could I be certain that her very-low-fat diet was the cause of her skin and hair problems? No, I could not. She had recently had a thorough physical, and no medical disorder had been diagnosed. So I ruled out that as a cause. What about perimenopause? She was thirty-eight, so it was possible. But it was an academic question, because the diet I put her on provided all the nutrients that her body required and regulated her blood sugar hormones. When she started to look better, she would also produce fewer stress hormones. My guess was that with her blood sugar and stress hormones in balance, she would not suffer symptoms from her ovarian hormones. But we would have to wait and see.

Jessica did not improve. It took a while for me to find out why. She finally admitted that she wasn't following my diet. She just couldn't bring herself to eat food that she knew contained fat. Jessica, like so many women her age, had been brainwashed for over a decade to view fat as the ultimate dietary demon. After several tries I finally convinced her that my Mediterranean clients had the best skin and hair I have ever seen. And all they used was vigin olive oil in cooking and on salads. Finally, the turning point was when her acquaintances began remarking on how much better she was looking, after she had grudgingly agreed to add olive oil to her salad dressing. I needed to say no more! Jessica was now well on her way to recovering youthful skin and hair.

Fats

Dietary fats provide the essential fatty acids required to produce hormones, they facilitate oxygen transportation, and they assist in the absorption of fat-soluble vitamins A, D, E, and K. Fats nourish our skin, nerves, and mucous membranes. They make food taste good and release the hormone cholecystokinin (CCK) from our stomach to send a message to our brain that we are no longer hungry. When there are not enough fats in our food, some or other of these bodily functions may not be performed satisfactorily.

Both dietary and body fats are made up of a combination of one to three fatty acids and a molecule of glycerol, an alcohol. Fats are called mono-, di-, or triglycerides, depending on the number of fatty acids in them. At least two fatty acids—linoleic acid and alpha-linolenic acid—are not made by the body and have to be obtained from food.

The terms *saturated* and *unsaturated* refer to the structure of the fat molecule. Saturated fats have all possible hydrogen atoms present, while unsaturated fats do not. Unsaturated fats are further classified as monounsaturated when they have one double bond between adjacent carbon atoms, and polyunsaturated when they have more. A simple way to tell the difference between them is that, at room temperature, saturated fats are solid and unsaturated fats are liquid. Contrary to popular opinion, unsaturated fats do not, as a general rule, have fewer calories than saturated fats. Most fats are a mixture of saturated, polyunsaturated, and monounsaturated, with one kind predominating.

Type of Fat	Room Temperature	Refrigerated
Saturated fats (except tropical oils)	Solid	Solid
Polyunsaturated fats	Liquid	Liquid (except when hydrogenated)
Monounsaturated fats	Liquid	Semisolid or solid

Oils are liquid fats, and omega-3,-6, and -9 oils are key suppliers of fatty acids to the body for the manufacture of important hormones. We will look at omega rich oils in the next chapter, (specifically flaxseed oil and evening primrose oil) that provide balm for female symptoms.

Food Sources of Saturated Fats

ANIMAL SOURCES

Pork, lamb, and beef fats
  (lard, tallow, and suet)
Organ meats

Full-fat dairy products
  (whole milk, cream cheese,
  ice cream, butter)

VEGETABLE SOURCES

Coconut oil
Cocoa butter

Palm oil
Palm kernel oil

Food Sources of Monounsaturated Fats

VEGETABLE, LEGUME, AND SEED SOURCES

Olive
Avocado
Almond
Apricot kernel

Peanut
Canola
High-oleic safflower and
  sunflower oils

Food Sources of Omega–3 Polyunsaturated Fats

ANIMAL SOURCES

Salmon
Mackerel
Herring
Cod
Sardines
Halibut
Tuna
Sablefish

Bass
Flounder
Anchovies
Trout
Crappie
Shrimp
Oysters

VEGETABLE SOURCES

Flaxseed oil
Pumpkinseed
Canola
Soybeans
Walnuts

Wheat germ
Wheat sprouts
Sea vegetables, fresh
Leafy greens

Food Sources of Omega–6 Polyunsaturated Fats

ANIMAL SOURCES

Mother's milk
Organ meats

Lean meats

VEGETABLE SOURCES

Safflower
Sunflower
Corn
Soy
Sesame

Nuts and seeds, raw
Legumes
Spirulina
Leafy greens

BOTANICALS

Borage
Evening primrose oil

Blackcurrant seed oil

Healthful and Unhealthful Fats

Some experts have begun asking if saturated fat is being blamed in an oversimplified way for high cholesterol levels and blocking of arteries. One viewpoint is that Americans eat too much saturated fat but that other people who eat monounsaturated fat have fewer cardiovascular problems. Italians and Greeks have been eating much the same diets, with high amounts of monounsaturated fat in the form of olive oil, for more than three thousand years. Their cardiovascular health is much better than ours, as is that of the French, who eat food rich in saturated fat (butter, cream, and liver patés) along with their red wine. Despite earlier reports, people in countries that use a lot of palm oil and coconut oil, both rich in saturated fat, don't have high rates of cardiovascular disease. And how do the Masai and some Eskimos live almost exclusively on saturated fat? Denouncing saturated fat as a public enemy is the easy way out. I believe that as yet only part of the story has been heard.

Hydrogenated vegetable fats are definitely worthy of suspicion for increasing health problems. Bubbling hydrogen gas through a liquid polyunsaturated fat causes more of the hydrogen sites on the molecules to become occupied and helps prevent the fat from becoming rancid. However, this hydrogenation process also makes the polyunsaturated fat more like a saturated fat in molecular structure, and no longer a natural form of food. The storekeeper gains longer shelf life for the product, and the customer loses with a less healthful food.

From 5 to 35 percent of the fat in hydrogenated vegetable oils (including margarine) may be composed of trans fatty acids. Our bodies did not evolve to process fatty acids with the trans molecular structure (a mirror image of the natural structure). Trans fatty acids are being connected with an increasing number of disorders and may interfere with the manufacture of hormones. Jane E. Brody reported in the *New York Times* that trans fatty acids have been linked to an increased risk of developing breast cancer. A study of nearly seven hundred postmenopausal European women showed that those whose bodies contained the highest levels of trans fatty acids were 40 percent more likely to develop breast cancer than those with the lowest levels. The study's lead researcher, Lenore Kohlmeier, professor of epidemiology and nutrition at the University of North Carolina at Chapel Hill, said that American women eat twice as much trans fatty acids as European women. Commercially baked bread, crackers, muffins, rolls, and biscuits are the foods highest in trans fats. When in 1990 McDonald's changed from using beef tallow to partially hydrogenated vegetable oil for frying, the percentage of fat that came from trans fatty acids in their french fries increased from 5 percent to between 42 and 48 percent.

About 30 percent of calories should be derived from fats for a hormone-regulating diet. Fats supply nine calories per gram. I want you to include—not exclude—these tasty and good-for-you sources of unprocessed quality fats and oils: flaxseed oil, olive oil, canola oil, nuts, seeds, and avocado.

Eicosanoids

The fat in our food provides our bodies with the essential fatty acids to build eicosanoids, hormones that control bodily functions. These hormones have lifetimes of less than a few seconds, and prostaglandins are the only ones most nutritionally conscious individuals recognize as a familiar name. Eicosanoids, according to some authorities, control just about all hormones and every bodily function. They are known to be affected by the nutrients that our bodies absorb from food.

Eicosanoids are assigned to "good" and "bad" categories. This is simply for convenience of discussion, because our bodies, to be healthy, need both categories in balance. Perhaps "positive" and "negative" would be better labels. Bad eicosanoids increase on a high-carbohydrate diet, with undesirable results in our bodies.

Eicosanoid Functions

Good Eicosanoids	Bad Eicosanoid
Blood vessel dilating	Blood vessel constricting
Anti-blood clotting	Pro-blood clotting
Bronchiole dilating	Bronchiole constricting
Anti-cell proliferation	Pro-cell proliferation
Immunity strengthening	Immunity weakening
Anti-inflaming	Proinflaming
Cholesterol reducing	Cholesterol increasing
Pain decreasing	Pain increasing
Antidepressive	—
Endocrine hormone stimulating	—
—	Triglycerides increasing

A Balanced Diet

Our food needs to be composed of a *balance* of carbohydrates, proteins, and fats. A stable blood sugar level is one of the benefits of a balanced diet. With a stable blood sugar level, a woman experiences fewer health risks and enjoys balanced moods, extended energy, and greater concentration and attention span.

We've all been hearing about a balanced diet since our schooldays, and I mention it here only because so many of us as adults ignore it. Eating a lot of junk food, as Americans do, is putting yourself at risk of an unbalanced diet. Fad diets that deprive your body of nutrients that it requires are certainly unbalanced. Carbo loading for high-performance sports is a deliberate but no less stressful and unhealthful way to unbalance a diet.

For hormonal regulation and sustained physical and mental effort, nothing beats a diet with an approximately 40/30/30 ratio. The Changing Diet uses this carbohydrates/protein/fats ratio as a base on which to build a hormone-regulating eating plan.

Chapter 5

Healing Oils

Lose Weight,
Up Your Mood, and
Lower Your Blood Pressure

W ithout sufficient quantities of two very special fatty acids, your body cannot manufacture all kinds of important substances, including the stress and ovarian hormones. If your very-low-fat diet does not supply enough omega–3 and –6 fatty acids for your body requirements, you can suffer serious damage to your health. Omega–3 fatty acids are found in the oils of cold-water fish, and certain vegetable, seed, and botanical oils are rich in omega–6 fatty acids.

In spite of their name, fatty acids are not themselves fats. They are the building blocks of fats, like amino acids are the building blocks of proteins. As mentioned in the last chapter, the human body can manufacture all but two of the fatty acids it needs. One of these essential fatty acids is an omega–3 fatty acid, and the other an omega–6. They have somewhat similar names, the omega–3 being called alpha-linolenic acid, and the omega–6, cis-linoleic acid. In the body, they break down into a series of compounds, most of which have equally confusing names.

The health benefits attributed to polyunsaturated fats are rightfully those of omega fatty acids. Along with the B-complex vitamins and vitamin E, the omegas control cell growth as well as help in the manufacture of hormones. Their byproducts are ingredients of cell membranes and nerve sheaths. These fatty acids help dissolve body fat, lowering blood levels of cholesterol and triglycerides. They distribute the fat-soluble vitamins A, D, E, and K through body tissues. And they are building blocks for prostaglandins.

Prostaglandins

I mentioned eicosanoids in the last chapter, the best-known kind of which are prostaglandins. Indeed, many use the names interchangeably, as I will do in this chapter for simplicity. You will remember that prostaglandins/eicosanoids are very short-lived (less than a few seconds), hormonelike substances that control most if not all of our bodily functions. The better-known endocrine hormones (insulin, progesterone) are secreted by glands, while prostaglandins seem to be secreted at locations all over the body and by various kinds of tissue.

Among many other functions, prostaglandins are known to stimulate the secretion of hormones and to alleviate various PMS and perimenopause symptoms.

From a nutritional point of view, some of the steps from an omega fatty acid to a prostaglandin are useful to know, because the intermediate substances are also available in food.

For the first step of the following transition of an omega–3 fatty acid to a prostaglandin, several things are required: vitamin B_6, magnesium, zinc, and insulin. EPA stands for eicosapentaenoic acid.

Alpha-linolenic acid (omega–3)
EPA
Prostaglandin E3

Alpha-linolenic acid (omega–3) is found in wheat sprouts, wheat germ, nuts, and seeds—and in their oils. Flaxseeds, soybeans, and walnuts—and their oils—are very rich in omega–3. EPA is found in large amounts in cold-water fish oils from fatty fish such as salmon, sardines, and mackerel. The fish should be fresh, because much of the EPA deteriorates in the freezing or canning process.

Cis-linoleic acid (an omega–6 fatty acid) can become a prostaglandin in two different ways. Again, vitamin B$_6$, magnesium, zinc, and insulin are required for the first step. GLA stands for gamma-linolenic acid. The step from GLA to prostaglandin E1 requires vitamins B$_3$ (niacin) and C.

Cis-linoleic acid (omega–6)
GLA
Prostaglandin E1

Cis-linoleic acid (omega–6)
GLA
Arachidonic acid
Prostaglandin E2

One hundred percent expeller-pressed and unrefined oils are the best source of cis-linoleic acid (omega–6). These oils are produced by pressing seeds, nuts, or vegetables through a screw press at the lowest possible temperatures. Solvents or chemicals are not used, and, unlike refined oils, an unrefined oil is not filtered a second time, deodorized, or bleached.

You can contribute ready-made GLA to both of the above processes by eating oils and plants that contain GLA, such as evening primrose oil, gooseberry oil, spirulina, and borage.

Partially hydrogenated vegetable oils and other commercially processed oils and margarine, along with fried food—what I call damaged fats—can interfere with the transformation of EPA or GLA into prostaglandins. Excess heat, air, light, or hydrogenation in the processing turns beneficial polyunsaturated fats into harmless substances. On a more general level, a bad diet or lifestyle habits, illness, or medication can interfere with the transition of fatty acids to prostaglandins.

Healing Benefits for Women

So many bodily functions, health benefits, and disorders are associated with the metabolism of essential fatty acids and prostaglandins that an entire book could be devoted to them. We will look at just a few health benefits of special concern to women in their thirties and forties.

- Essential fatty acids, through the prostaglandins they help manufacture, are a prime source of relief from many perimenopausal symptoms.

- Fish oils containing EPA lower blood cholesterol and triglyceride levels and reduce the stickiness of blood platelets, thereby lowering the risk of blood clots.

- Prostaglandin E3 relaxes blood vessel walls, preventing arterial spasms and lowering blood pressure. Migraine symptoms may be relieved in this way.

- For women who are diabetic or borderline, lack of insulin may interfere with the manufacture of EPA or GLA, resulting in a shortage of prostaglandins and symptoms of nerve twitching, infection, and sexual dysfunction. Ingesting oils rich in EPA or GLA may make up for the deficiency.

- Skin, hair, and nails benefit from GLA or EPA in combination with zinc and vitamin A. My clients have noticed an improved complexion, strengthened nails, and a disappearance of dandruff. Eczema, acne, and psoriasis show improvement, too.

- Even if you do nothing else in the way of diet and exercise, you can lose up to five pounds by regularly using omega oils as salad dressing.

○ The omega fatty acids combat depression. They also help with hangovers and alcohol withdrawal symptoms—and we all know someone who could use this kind of assistance.

○ The essential fatty acids make cell membranes less permeable to the passage of yeast and thus check the spread of infection.

○ Fish oils cause tissue changes that may lower the risk of breast cancer. John Glaspy and colleagues at the Jonsson Center of the University of California at Los Angeles put twenty-five American women on a diet that mimicked the foods, including fish oils, eaten by Asian women, who have a much lower rate of breast cancer than American women. The fish oil capsules in this diet caused a beneficial rise in the concentration of fatty acids in tissue, which is expected to lower the likelihood of breast cancer.

Food Sources of Omega Fatty Acids

From many studies, it appears that American women do not ingest enough omega-3 fatty acids for their general health needs, let alone enough to alleviate female symptoms. While the majority of American women seem to get enough omega-6 fatty acids, if they are derived from processed or hydrogenated oils, these fatty acids are biochemically impotent. The inescapable conclusion is that women in their thirties and forties need a kind of food plan resembling the Changing Diet, which is rich in both omega-3 and -6 food sources. And if the Changing Diet is not sufficient to fully cure their symptoms, they need additional omega-rich foods or supplements.

Comparison of American and Asian diets raises the question of the correct proportion in which to ingest the two essential fatty acids. Taking too much of either of these omega fatty acids alone can cause imbalances. Since the American diet is clearly lacking in omega-3, it makes sense to increase omega-3 over omega-6. I recommended a 2:1 ratio in favor of omega-3 for three to nine months to build up body reserves, and after that a 1:1 ratio.

Mother's milk supplies adequate quantities of both omega-3 and -6 fatty acids and is one of the few foods to do so. Cow's milk is a comparatively poor source, and skim milk even poorer. To seek additional quantities of the two essential fatty acids in our diet, we need to look at different food sources for each. A noteworthy exception to this is flaxseed oil, which contains both.

Omega-3/EPA Food Sources

Regular meals of cold-water fish and seafoods provide enough EPA for ordinary health needs but may not be sufficient to alleviate perimenopausal symptoms. The amounts eaten on the Changing Diet should be sufficient to remedy milder symptoms. If your symptoms are stronger, you need to deliberately seek out omega-3 and -6 or EPA and GLA food sources and supplements.

Flaxseed oil is the richest source of the omega-3 essential fatty acid alpha-linolenic acid, the precursor of EPA.

Percentage of Alpha-Linolenic Acid (Omega-3), Precursor of EPA, by Total Weight of Seeds

Flaxseed	8-60%
Chia seed	0%
Hemp seed	0%
Pumpkinseed (Eastern European type)	5%
Canola oil	0%
Soybean oil	8%
American black walnut	5%
Leafy vegetables, fresh (average serving)	0.009%

North Atlantic sardine oil, at 18 percent EPA, is the richest food source of EPA. This, of course, is not the oil that sardines are canned in, but an oil made from the fish themselves. Salmon oil has 9 percent EPA, and mackerel oil about 5 percent. The fish get their EPA from eating shrimplike krill, which in turn eat cold-water plankton, which use EPA as a kind of antifreeze—plankton in warmer waters are less rich in EPA. In general, the oilier the fish flesh, the more EPA it contains.

Sea vegetables (edible seaweed) and green leafy vegetables are also sources of EPA.

EPA Content in 3.5-Ounce Servings of Various Fish

Fish	EPA, milligrams
Anchovy	747
Chinook salmon	633
Herring	606
Mackerel	585
Albacore tuna	337
Pacific halibut	194
Atlantic cod	93
Rainbow trout	84
Haddock	72
Swordfish	30
Red snapper	19
Sole	10

Fish Oil Capsules

Many of us don't get the opportunity frequently to eat fresh cold-water fish with oily flesh, and a lot of us also aren't exactly looking forward to eating fish anyway. Besides, fish with high fat contents are most likely to have fat-soluble toxins in their flesh, such as PCBs, mercury, and arsenic. Fish oil capsules, while they may not deliver as much EPA as the highest-rated fish in a fresh state, certainly make up for it in convenience. But the capsule oils need to be of high quality, purity, and freshness. I use three tests to ensure that they are:

1. **Taste.** Puncture a capsule with a pin and squeeze a drop of oil onto your tongue. A pure, high-quality fish oil does not taste fishy. A fresh oil tastes mild and sweet. Rancid oil tastes bitter.

2. **Color and clarity.** Light color and clearness indicate fresh-ness and lack of PCB or heavy metal contamination. As fish oil ages, it darkens and becomes cloudy.

3. **Freezability.** Put a capsule in the freezer compartment of your refrigerator. If its contents congeal within a few hours, it has a high saturated fat content. The higher a capsule's satu-rated fat content, the lower its EPA content.

Omega–6/GLA Food Sources

Unrefined vegetable oils are the richest food source of cis-linoleic acid, the precursor of GLA. Other foods rich in this essential fatty acid are green leafy vegetables (such as kale, collard greens, and Swiss chard), liver, kidneys, brains, sweetbreads, and lean red meat. Flaxseed oil is 18 to 20 percent omega–6.

Richest Sources of Cis-Linoleic Acid (Omega–6), Precursor of GLA

UNREFINED

Vegetable Oil	Linoleic Acid, %
Safflower	78
Sunflower	69
Corn	62
Soy	61
Walnut	59
Cottonseed	54
Sesame	43
Rice bran	32
Peanut	31
Olive	15
Coconut	2

Richest Sources of GLA

Borage plant	24%
Black currant oil	15–19%
Gooseberry oil	10–12%
Evening primrose oil	2–9%

Flaxseed Oil

Popular vegetable oils like olive, sunflower, almond, safflower, avocado, sesame, peanut, and corn, while containing varying amounts of omega–6, contain negligible omega–3. Of the readily available vegetable oils, only three contain both omega–3 and –6 essential fatty acids. They are as follows:

Oil	Omega–3	Omega–6
Flaxseed oil	58–60%	18–20%
Canola oil	10%	24%
Soy oil	8%	50%

Since omega–3 is low or even nonexistent in the American diet, flaxseed oil, with its high percentage of omega–3 and medium percentage of omega–6, is by far the most desirable vegetable oil. It came into prominence through Johanna Budwig's successful use of it with milk as a tumor-reducing medication in Germany in the 1950s. She recommended that one or two tablespoons of low-fat cottage cheese be ingested with the flaxseed oil to provide sulfur-containing amino acids to interact with it in the body.

Quite apart from its qualities as a remedy for perimenopausal symptoms, flaxseed oil has a reputation as a cancer fighter. This is due to its ability to counteract the cancer-causing abilities of some omega–6 fatty acids. It's believed that some prostaglandins derived from arachidonic acid (see the second of the two omega–6 chemical transitions earlier in this chapter) are cancer promoters. EPA and another omega–3 fatty acid, docosahexaenoic acid (DHA), compete with and displace arachidonic acid in cell membranes. In this way, these omega–3 fatty acids protect the body, particularly against cancers of the breast, colon, throat, and skin. Flaxseed oil is also credited with a long list of other health benefits, including lowering blood cholesterol levels, helping insulin receptor binding, boosting the immune system, and bettering mineral metabolism.

Author, nutritionist, and research pharmacist Ross Pelton claims that the imbalance in our diet between omega–3 and –6 fatty acids is responsible for many of our growing health problems. He points out that hydrogenation and refining of vegetable oils and processing of grains have caused an 80 percent reduction of omega–3 fatty acids in the American diet over the past hundred years. While Pelton is talking about the incidence of cancer, I have seen a similar effect in perimenopausal symptoms. When women with symptoms restored the balance of omega–3 and –6 fatty acids in their bodies, their symptoms evaporated.

Because the Changing Diet already includes omega–3-rich foods such as fresh cold-water fish and both flaxseed and canola oils in the menu planner and recipes, many of my clients on this diet have found that taking an additional tablespoon of flaxseed oil a day is sufficient to get their bodies back in balance. Women not on the Changing Diet need to take two tablespoons a day. When buying flaxseed oil, try to get the kind that is high in lig-

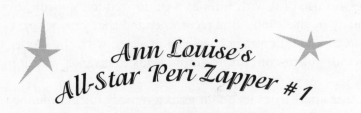

Ann Louise's
All-Star Peri Zapper #1

Flaxseed Oil

As an all-around peri balancer—especially for skin conditions, depression, and fatigue—nothing beats a daily tablespoonful of flaxseed oil that is high in lignans. Swallow as is or use as a salad dressing or topping for grains and veggies and in no-heat recipes.

nans. Lignans are a class of phytonutrients that quell perimenopause symptoms, as well as quenching free radicals and
combating the cell-proliferating powers of excess estrogen. The
lignans occur in the fibrous shell of the flaxseed and therefore are
liable to be almost absent from ordinary flaxseed oil. In oils high
in lignans, tiny particles (called particulate) of lignan-containing
seed husk are held in suspension in the oil.

Flaxseed oil has a nutty flavor. People who don't care for this
taste, or for the consistency of the oil, can swallow it quickly and
wash it down with tea or some other drink. Because heat, light,
and oxygen quickly cause the oil to become rancid, it should be
purchased only in a black, opaque bottle, which should be refrigerated after being opened. Obviously, it should not be used in
cooking or baking, although it can be poured on hot food.
Flaxseed oil can be found in almost all health food stores.

Take one or two tablespoons daily, as a salad dressing or driz-
zled over any side dish, such as baked potato or steamed vegetables or grains.

Evening Primrose Oil

Evening primrose oil, a Native American traditional remedy, has a
wonderfully easing effect on a broad array of perimenopause
symptoms. In a study at St. Thomas's Hospital in London, of the
women with breast tenderness taking evening primrose oil, 72
percent found relief. Women also find it good for mood changes,
anxiety, irritability, headaches, and fluid retention. These healing
powers are due at least in part to its ability to regulate prostaglandins. A source of GLA, evening primrose oil also has a number
of other health benefits, including its ability to combat inflamma-
tion, hardening of the arteries, and heart disease.

Some of my clients claim that *nothing else* that I recommend
eases their symptoms as well as evening primrose oil. My explanation for this is that much of the GLA in commercial vegetable
oils, even those that are of high quality and unrefined, probably
gets damaged in the processing and storage of the product. This
interferes with the GLA's ability to interact with other substances.
Certainly, there's no doubt that evening primrose oil GLA is

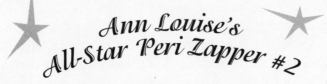

Ann Louise's
All-Star Peri Zapper #2

Evening Primrose Oil

For breast tenderness, particularly, but also for mood changes, anxiety, irritability, headaches, and water retention, take two capsules (500 milligrams) of evening primrose oil twice daily after food.

---

much more biologically active than GLA from commercial vegetable oils.

In the London study, although a few women took evening primrose oil every day, most started taking it three days before they expected their symptoms to occur and continued until the start of their period. They took two capsules twice daily after food. In a few cases of very severe symptoms, women took three capsules twice daily. Some women took vitamin B_6 at the same time.

Olive Oil

People around the shores of the Mediterranean have been using olive oil as a nutrient from the times of the Bible and ancient Greece and Rome. Although it has no omega–3 fatty acids and only 8 percent omega–6 fatty acids, this monounsaturated oil has countless health benefits, not all of which are known even after three thousand years. Many nutritionists would not be surprised if future research uncovers that olive oil does indeed help alleviate a number of perimenopausal symptoms. It's already known that the oleic acid in olive oil helps prevent the spread of yeast infections. And olive oil is a preventive of breast cancer. In a study of Greek women conducted by Harvard's School of Public Health and published in the January 1995 *Journal of the National Cancer*

Institute, women who consume olive oil more than once a day were found to have a 25 percent reduction in their chance of getting breast cancer.

Olive oil comes in three grades: extra virgin, virgin, and pure. The first two grades are pressed from a single pressing without heat and are therefore desirable. The differences between these two grades lie in the quality of olives used. Pure olive oil is a combination of refined oils from later pressings and is much inferior.

Canola Oil

Derived from rapeseed, canola oil, introduced fairly recently, has 62 percent monounsaturated fat in comparison to olive oil's 77 percent. It is also the oil lowest in saturated fat. Fat phobia was at its peak at the time of the introduction of canola oil in the mid-80's, and its low saturated fat content was regarded as a major health advance in consumer products. Canola oil remains an attractive alternative to olive oil today because it is tasteless. But canola has another major advantage from my point of view, in that it has 10 percent omega–3 fatty acids and 24 percent omega–6.

The Essential Woman

Some of us love to shop around, mixing and matching various nutrients to suit our bodies individual needs. But more of us wish that all these nutrients had more user-friendly names, were a lot less complicated, and could all be taken in one magic spoonful. With this in mind, I specially formulated a healing oil for women in their thirties and forties.

This oil, called "the Essential Woman," is not magic and does not contain all the nutrients a woman needs; that would not be possible! What it does contain are the essential fatty acids that we have been discussing in this chapter, along with other symptom-alleviating nutrients that will be discussed in later chapters.

The Essential Woman Healing Oil*

* Manufactured exclusively by Barlean's Organic Oils. Product of U.S.A.

INGREDIENTS:

Organic flaxseed oil, evening primrose oil, flaxseed particulate, isoflavones, saponins, and protease inhibitors isolated from soy

ONE TABLESPOON PROVIDES APPROXIMATELY:

Fatty Acids

Omega–3	4300 mg
Omega–6	2455 mg
Omega–9	1360 mg
Evening primrose oil	1000 mg

Lignans

Secoisolariciresinol diglycoside/matairesinol	6 mg

Isoflavones

Diadzein	22 mg
Genistein	8 mg
Glycitein	15 mg

Other

Flaxseed particulate	2660 mg
Saponins	60 mg
Rosemary/ascorbic acid	20 mg
Protease inhibitors	9 mg

Some of the ingredients of this healing oil will be familiar to readers of this chapter. Others may require a brief comment. The main omega–9 fatty acid is oleic acid, which is mainly found in olive oil, high-oleic safflower and sunflower oils, and avocado oil and to a lesser extent in almond, apricot kernel, canola, peanut, and sesame oils. Oleic acid combats the spread of yeast infections. Isoflavones, found naturally in beans, peas, and lentils, help relieve female symptoms, block estrogen's cancer-promoting ability, and inactivate enzymes produced by cancer cells. Saponins are antioxidants and lower cholesterol. Rosemary, an astringent herb, alleviates migraine, is an antioxidant, and combats heart disease and infections. Protease inhibitors, from soy, limit the rate of cell growth, block cancer cell enzymes, and assist cells in repairing DNA damage. Quite a lot in a single spoonful of oil!

The suggested dosage is one tablespoon daily. You may swallow a spoonful of the oil, mix it with low-fat yogurt or cottage cheese, use it as a salad dressing, or put it in oatmeal, a protein drink, or a blended beverage. I love it on air-popped popcorn!

After opening, the bottle should be kept refrigerated. For storage, freezing will extend the shelf life of the oil approximately three months beyond the "best before" date marked on the bottle.

Other healthful oil products that I can recommend are the following:

Omega Twin Hi Lignan, from Barlean's

Flax Oil Hi Lignan, from Barlean's

MaxEPA, from Solgar

Eskimo 3, from Cardinova

Omega–3 Fish Oil Concentrate, from Dale Alexander

Super Omega–3, Norwegian Salmon Oil, and Evening Primrose Oil, from Carlson

Chapter 6

Vitamins and Minerals

*Zapping Anxiety, Insomnia,
Bloating, Nervousness,
and Irritability*

The vitamins and minerals discussed in this chapter are those that have special significance for perimenopause symptoms. Symptoms such as anxiety, insomnia, bloating, nervousness, and irritability are often results of low tissue levels of a vitamin or mineral. When you take an oral supplement, the symptoms can often diminish and finally vanish. Two kinds of mineral imbalance are often the cause of symptoms—zinc-copper and magnesium-calcium.

The good news about symptoms that are caused by vitamin or mineral deficiencies is that they can usually be brought under control through some simple dietary changes and by taking the proper dietary supplements.

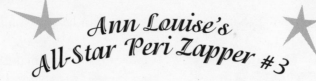

M 'n' M (Multivitamins and Magnesium)

Many women's perimenopause symptoms (such as mood swings, insomnia, anxiety, tissue dryness, and water retention) are alleviated by the following combination of supplements:

- Vitamin B complex, including 50 to 100 milligrams of vitamin B_6
- Vitamin C, 1000 milligrams three times a day
- Vitamin E, 400 to 1200 international units
- Magnesium, 500 to 1000 milligrams before sleeping

When you feel that your hormones are back in better balance, you may be able to cut back to 1000 milligrams a day of vitamin C and to 400 international units of vitamin E.

Michelle

Having seen me interviewed on a television show, Michelle found my phone number and called for an appointment. She said she was forty-four and getting married for a second time. As her wedding day neared, she was aware that the occasional bloating from which she had been suffering for some years was becoming more frequent. Naturally, this upset her. Even her eyelids, she said, were now becoming puffy, and she seemed to be developing breathing difficulties. She was afraid it was becoming a permanent condition. I had spoken about bloating and water retention on the TV program. Could I help her?

When Michelle came to my office a few days later, I saw that she was visibly bloated. Other than that, she had an attractive appearance, with a warm, sensitive manner, and was casually dressed in a T-shirt and faded blue jeans.

When I questioned her intensely about her medical history and lifestyle, as I do all my clients, she told me that a doctor had prescribed pills for her condition a couple of years previously. The pills, whose name she could not recall, eased the bloating but left her skin dry and scaly, so she had stopped taking them. Michelle was vague about her eating habits. She seemed to eat at no fixed times and often mentioned brand-name fast foods.

The pills had probably caused important nutrients to be excreted with her excess fluid, and this had resulted in her dry, scaly skin. The doctor might have recommended that she take supplements with the pills, but Michelle didn't recall this.

From her irregular eating habits and fondness for fast food, I guessed that she might have a vitamin deficiency, as do so many people with that lifestyle. I recommended that she take a multivitamin pill every day, plus a B-50 complex pill once a day and an additional 50 milligrams of vitamin B_6.

Vitamin B_6 proved to be what she needed. After her bloating subsided, I reduced the dosage and had her take the B_6 as part of the once-a-day B-50 complex supplement. This was enough to prevent furthur recurrences. Although I don't believe that she ever completely abandoned junk food, Michelle did make other improvements in her diet, including eating adequate meals on a regular schedule.

But was this perimenopause or simply a vitamin deficiency that could have occurred at any age? In her case, I can't say for sure, but I can tell you what I suspect. I believe that, had she stayed on her vitamin-deficient diet, in due course her B_6 deficiency would have been joined by other deficiencies, possibly in magnesium or zinc, and she would have developed other unpleasant symptoms. Women in their late thirties and forties tend to display symptoms from years of unhealthful eating. Such symptoms would be indistinguishable from perimenopause symptoms. We know that symptoms result much more often from multiple risk factors than from single causes. We could think of perimenopause and a vitamin deficiency as separate risk factors that combined in Michelle's case to produce the symptom of bloating.

Vitamin B₆

Vitamin B_6 (pyridoxine) has often been called a "woman's guardian angel" because of its power to relieve perimenopausal symptoms, particularly water retention and bloating, skin eruptions, mood swings, and even depression and anxiety. High concentrations of B_6 increase the synthesis of the neurotransmitter dopamine and inhibit secretion of the milk-stimulating hormone prolactin. This alleviates anxiety, irritability, mood swings, and nervous tension. Vitamin B_6 reduces levels of estrogen and elevates progesterone levels. Additionally, B_6 helps balance tissue levels of magnesium, a mineral noted for its ability to alleviate perimenopause symptoms.

Vitamin B_6 is needed for normal secretion of serotonin, the brain neurotransmitter that regulates mood, pain, sleep, and appetite. This vitamin has been shown to improve memory, particularly long-term memory, and increases the brain's capacity to store information.

While B_6 is probably effective on its own, most nutritionists agree that since the B vitamins affect the absorption and metabolism of one another, B_6 should be taken with B-complex vitamins. From the early 1940s, lack of B vitamins has been known to be responsible for women's health problems. Pioneer endocrinologist in women's health Guy Abraham emphasized that a woman's liver needs a complete array of B vitamins to change excess estrogen into its metabolically useful form.

Dr. Leo Galland found that most women with yeast infections have problems metabolizing B_6 and are therefore deficient in this vitamin. Taking contraceptive pills increases the body's need for B_6 and thus can cause a deficiency. Vitamin B_6 is important for collagen formation and bone strength later in life, due to its role in amino acid metabolism. Dr. John M. Ellis says that B_6 helps prevent and control nausea and toxemia during pregnancy. Recently, a lack of this vitamin has been connected to carpal tunnel syndrome.

Food sources of B_6 include soybeans, kale, spinach, bananas, liver, nuts, whole grains, meat, fish, poultry, legumes, sunflower seeds, avocados, and green peppers.

Michelle's total dosage of 100 milligrams a day was recommended for a limited time for her water retention. Your daily dosage to prevent perimenopause symptoms should range from 50 to 100 milligrams per day, spread out over the day. A full B-complex vitamin should be taken with the B_6.

Vitamin E

Itchy skin, a susceptibility to infections, and varicose veins are all symptoms of low levels of vitamin E in your body. For perimenopausal women, vitamin E is a marvelous remedy for vaginal dryness, hot flashes, breast tenderness, and fibrocystic breasts, in dosages ranging from 400 to 1200 international units per day. Interestingly, many experts feel that, at the cellular level, vitamin E is molecularly similar to estrogen and therefore functions as a natural hormone replacement! Vitamin E suppositories and ointments dramatically soothe vaginal dryness. For women generally, this vitamin promotes heart health, good skin, and overall physical and emotional well-being.

The vitamin's natural food sources are vegetable oils, nuts, and seeds. Diets that eliminate these fatty foods can cause low levels of vitamin E. Beverly Hills nutritionist Evelyn Tribole told *The Walking Magazine* that she considers it difficult to meet the RDA for vitamin E while sticking to a low-fat diet. Unless we eat the fatty foods rich in this vitamin, most of us need a supplement.

Women who consumed as little as 5 to 8 international units of vitamin E a day cut their risk of dying of heart disease by 30 percent, according to a study conducted by Dr. Lawrence Kushi at the University of Minnesota. And women who consumed more than 8 international units a day cut their risk by 60 percent!

Iron

Iron is an ingredient of hemoglobin, and you can become anemic through loss of iron-rich blood in menstruation. When you have iron-deficiency anemia, you feel tired and cold all the time and have listless hair, pale dry skin, and dark circles under your eyes.

Lethargy, lack of concentration, headaches, and irritability can be symptoms also. Heavy physical exercise, pregnancy, or nursing significantly increases your need for iron. Perhaps four out of every five women who are very active physically ingest inadequate amounts of iron.

Iron deficiency can cause eating disorders. David L. Watts, Ph.D., director of research at Trace Elements, Inc., in Dallas, once described a woman patient with a bizarre eating disorder due to iron deficiency. Called pica, the disorder involves an abnormal craving to eat substances other than food. His patient's craving was for paper. Her craving began gradually, without any specific cause that she could remember. Her appetite for paper increased until it became uncontrollable. If she became emotionally moved as she read a book, she ate the pages. She ate the wrappers as well as the candy inside. When she used a tissue, she couldn't use just one—she ate the whole boxful, and then the box. Yet her cure was simple and completely successful: oral iron supplements.

Iron deficiency can interfere with the proper functioning of your thyroid gland. An amino acid that is converted to the precursor of the thyroid hormone thyroxine is reduced by 50 percent in iron-deficient women. Because of the close relationship of the thyroid gland to the adrenal glands, they may be affected, too.

Increased secretion of your parathyroid hormone can also result in iron deficiency. This takes place because the parathyroid hormone increases your body's absorption of calcium, which is antagonistic to the absorption of iron.

While it is desirable for active women who are still menstruating to take an iron supplement, you need to keep in mind that iron is double-edged. Too little can cause anemia, and too much can result in the far more undesirable conditions of heart disease and cancer. Iron overload can also be caused from a genetic disorder known as hemochromatosis, a condition said to affect one in every three hundred Americans. Women are much more likely to have too much iron after they stop menstruating. The association of too much iron with heart disease brings up an interesting possibility. Because women's rate of heart disease starts to equal that of men after menopause, estrogen has been thought to be the protective factor in preventing heart disease in women before menopause. This may not be true. The real protective factor may be the monthly loss of iron-rich blood. Obviously, if you no longer menstruate regularly, you should not take iron supplements. I suggest that as soon as you stop menstruating, start monitoring your ferritin level, which measures the iron stored in your body. You do this through a blood test on visits to your doctor. In this way, you can assess whether iron buildup is a problem you need to be concerned about. If tests indicate that you have iron buildup, you will need to avoid iron-rich foods and multivitamins to which iron has been added.

The best food sources for iron are dark green leafy vegetables, beans, beets, eggs, molasses, wheat germ, dried fruit, liver, and red meat. For perimenopause symptoms, you need 15 milligrams of iron a day, if you are menstruating regularly. Pregnant women need twice that. You'll find that taking vitamin C dramatically increases your body's absorption of iron. Red wine and dark beer also increase iron absorption. On the other hand, antacids, aspirin, caffeine, and some food preservatives interfere with iron absorption.

RDAs of Some Important Vitamins and Minerals During Perimenopause*

*Remember that RDAs were established to prevent deficiency, and do not necessarily represent the amounts needed for optimal health.

Vitamin B$_6$	1.6 milligrams
Vitamin E	12 international units
Iron	15 milligrams
Zinc	12 milligrams
Magnesium	280 milligrams
Calcium	1000 milligrams

Zinc-Copper Imbalance

Zinc is of particular importance to perimenopausal women for bone formation. This mineral assists in the absorption of vitamin D and is essential for osteoblast and osteoclast formation. Research studies on women of various ages have shown that zinc supplements help slow bone loss as well as boost compromised immune systems. Zinc supplements have recently been shown to fend off certain viruses, including the common cold. If you have low tissue levels of zinc, you are more likely to have perimenopause symptoms.

Tissue mineral analysis from hair has revealed that women with low zinc levels are likely to have high copper levels. In general, women in perimenopause tend to be copper-heavy and zinc-deficient. Zinc is closely associated with progesterone. When the level of zinc rises or falls, so does progesterone. Likewise, copper levels seem to rise or fall in tandem with estrogen levels. So we can say that perimenopausal women tend to be both progesterone- and zinc-deficient. Although these same women usually have too much copper in their tissues, and tend to be estrogen dominant. If their progesterone levels were adequate, their progesterone would counteract the effects of the estrogen and they would not have symptoms. Raising your zinc level with supplements and lowering your copper level through dietary vigilance could be the practical solution you are looking for.

Possible Symptoms from Low Zinc/ High Copper Ratio

Frontal headache	Food cravings
Heavy menstrual flow	Mood swings
Menstrual irregularities	Fatigue
Constipation	Depression
Weight gain	Yeast infections

The interesting thing is that low zinc/high copper symptoms are shared by perimenopause and copper toxicity. You can blame either one without ever being sure which is actually responsible or whether they are jointly responsible. Controlling the nutritional imbalance may be enough to cure the symptoms. But all too often, I have to convince clients that symptoms like menstrual irregularities, which they associate exclusively with female hormones, can have both a nutritional source and a nutritional cure.

In discussing zinc-to-copper ratios and similar matters, we need to keep in mind how the human metabolism varies from person to person. What upsets one woman goes unnoticed by another. Needless to say, the fact that one woman doesn't experience any symptoms doesn't make those symptoms any less real for the woman who does. In addition to personal differences in metabolism, other factors in our individual lifestyles can make us more prone to certain symptoms. For example, vegetarians in general are more likely to have copper overload and consequent perimenopause symptoms.

What causes a zinc deficiency to develop? First and foremost, stress. The next most common cause is a diet rich in sugar and processed carbohydrates. After that come vegetarian diets that omit meat and eggs, both good sources of zinc. Medications are a common cause. For instance, antidepressants, diuretics, and anti-inflammatory medications such as cortisone and Prednisone suppress your body's absorption of zinc, speed its excretion, or interfere with synergistic nutrients such as vitamin B_6 and magnesium. Alcohol is another cause of zinc deficiency, by increasing the excretion of the mineral through the kidneys. Grains, especially those in unleavened bread, have high levels of phytates. The phytic acid in such food binds with zinc and makes it impossible for your body to absorb it. The high fiber in vegetarian diets also causes zinc deficiency.

Too much zinc in your body, on the other hand, causes bad cholesterol (LDL) levels to rise and good cholesterol (HDL) levels to drop.

Tissue mineral analysis of hair samples is an excellent measure of zinc content in your body over time. However, neither tissue mineral analysis of hair nor the more traditional blood tests can reliably spot an acute zinc deficiency right now. The only reliable way to detect an acute deficiency, in my opinion, is through a person's positive response to zinc supplements.

Food sources for zinc include red meat, eggs, seafood, and whole grains. Vegetarians should definitely consider taking zinc supplements! If you have perimenopause symptoms, you need zinc supplements amounting to 15 to 50 milligrams per day.

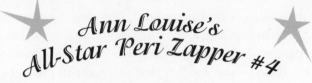

Ann Louise's
All-Star Peri Zapper #4

Think Zinc

Zinc (15 to 50 milligrams a day) helps to lower estrogen and increase progesterone levels, build strong bones, and keep your immune system in tiptop shape to ward off viruses. A must for vegetarians, whose diet is often lacking in this vital mineral.

Where does the copper come from? According to Dr. Paul C. Eck, diminished activity of the adrenal glands is probably the most important physiological cause of high copper levels. Adrenal gland activity is required to stimulate production of ceruloplasmin, the leading copper-binding protein. With diminished adrenal activity, the liver makes less ceruloplasmin and unbound copper starts to gather in various tissues and organs. Tissue mineral analysis shows that 70 to 80 percent of women have weak adrenal glands. Other sources of copper include the following:

- The mineral occurs naturally in drinking water in some parts of the country and may be added as copper sulfate to municipal drinking water and swimming pools to eradicate fungi, including yeast.

- Vitamin and mineral supplements often contain copper at levels harmful to some women.

- Vegetarian diets, high-soy diets, shellfish, organ meats, wheat germ and bran, corn oil, yeast, margarine, and mushrooms are all rich in copper.

- Copper water pipes and cookware are sources present in most American homes.

○ Birth control pills and copper intrauterine devices supply copper to the body, as do dental fillings, crowns, and other dental appliances.

○ People who work with metal, such as plumbers and welders, are at risk of absorbing toxic levels of copper.

Some Foods with a High Copper Content, in Milligrams per a Hundred Grams

Oysters	17.14
Lamb liver	5.60
Yeast, dried	4.98
Tea, bag	4.80
Cocoa powder	3.57
Soybeans	1.17
Curry powder	1.07

If you feel that you are overconsuming copper in foods, it is important for you to find supplements that are free of this mineral. With this requirement in mind, I formulated a copper-free, hypoallergenic multiple vitamin, mineral, glandular, and herbal product, called the Uni Key Female Multiple (available from Uni Key Health Systems at 1–800–888–4353).

Corinne

Having run twice in the New York marathon and once each in the Boston and London marathons, Corinne was a walking—or should I say running?—encyclopedia of sports information: sports injuries, high-performance nutrition recipes, sports superstitions, names of runners who took steroids, herbal infusions for stamina, and much, much more. I listened to her, enthralled and entertained, though sometimes appalled at what athletes believe. Much of her information was good, but some of it was misinterpreted, and sometimes dangerously so. An African American who worked in the computer field, she was tall and broad shouldered but with a narrow waist and long legs. She moved gracefully and was also athletically fit. She had a keen mind and, like many successful athletes, was a cool observer of her body. At thirty-nine, she was still running nine or ten kilometers regularly, but nothing longer because of her work schedule and lack of time for more extensive training.

Now something was wrong, she said. Corinne had been to a physician, who had told her she was developing osteoarthritis. She told the doctor that she suspected it had something to do with her extreme jumpiness.

"Yesterday," she said, "a friend dropped a plate on my kitchen floor and it shattered on the tiles just behind me. I got such a scare from the sound, you'd imagine I'd been in an earthquake. Then I got mad at her. It was only a dime store plate, but I felt so furious at her I had to step out in the backyard to avoid cussing her out over that little thing. I managed to control myself yesterday. But I don't always manage, I'm sorry to say." She took a breath and went on, "Now, I told things like that to the doctor and said if I was getting osteoarthritis, it had something to do with me leaping a foot in the air when someone drops a pin!"

"What did the doctor say?" I asked.

"She said I was only thirty-eight—as I was then—and so it was too early for my hormones to be causing it. Then she went on about how many athletes, when they feel their bodies aging, have an emotional crisis. I kind of yelled at her, I guess, that I'd never been a professional athlete or even won a big race and had already made adjustments for career and aging without going bananas. Several months passed, and then one day I was running around the reservoir in Central Park on a visit to New York, telling my sad story to this Columbia student I had met a few times previously. She told me what you say about magnesium. So here I am." She gave me a big smile. "I didn't run here. I flew."

I asked if the doctor had run a serum calcium test. She had. The results showed that Corinne's blood level of calcium was lower than normal. Corinne then decided to load up on calcium-rich foods like broccoli, turnip greens, and bok choy, only to find, on a retest, that her calcium level still remained low. Her level of 8.2 reminded me of my own levels years ago when I went out of my way to load up on calcium-rich foods (such as low-fat cheese and yogurt) and found that my blood level of the mineral still remained low, despite my calcium-rich dietary intake. Hearing of my own experience, Corinne agreed to have a tissue mineral analysis, which showed the exact opposite of her blood test. Her hair sample showed an excessively high amount of calcium in her tissues, which suggested to me that Corinne did not have a clinical calcium deficiency but was unable to use the excess calcium already present in her tissues (a situation that paralleled my own).

At the same time, she had a low tissue level of magnesium. Based on her report and on the lab recommendations, I suggested that she eat magnesium-rich foods (such as greens, almonds, and beans) and try 500 to 1000 milligrams of magnesium daily until she took another blood test and tissue mineral analysis in two months' time. Her blood level of calcium had risen from 8.2 to 9.0, and tissue mineral analysis from a hair sample revealed that her tissue level of calcium was now normal, even though she was not taking any calcium supplements and no longer was eating calcium-rich foods.

The high calcium content of the foods that she had been eating when she came to see me at first was not being absorbed into her bones because of a lack of magnesium, and the excess calcium in her tissues was affecting her nerves and contributing to her osteoarthritis.

Because, as I said, athletes are such objective reporters on their bodily conditions, I asked her to send me frequent reports on her progress. Her nerves are much better and she seems to be warding off her osteoarthritis. From a newspaper clipping she sent, I saw that she was the first woman across the finish line in a California race earlier this year.

Magnesium-Calcium Imbalance

You are constantly being advised, in television and print media, to drink milk and eat low-fat yogurt, cheese, and other dairy products to build your bones and avoid osteoporosis. According to the ads and advice, the calcium and vitamin D that these products contain will protect you from becoming a frail-boned woman who falls and breaks her hip. It's not quite that simple, because your body has a say in all this. Calcium is one of the least understood nutrients. The vast majority of American women do not have a true calcium deficiency. But they do have an inability to utilize the excess calcium that is already in their tissues.

Our bodies are not much different biochemically from those of our Stone Age ancestors forty thousand years ago. We could live very healthily today on the diet they ate. The only calcium-rich food they had was mother's milk. Animals were domesticated only ten thousand years ago. For thirty thousand years, at least, our ancestors managed to get along without dairy products. Why do we need them now? As you may have guessed, we don't—or at least not in the quantities that the ads suggest.

One good reason for not needing dairy products is that the majority of people over four years old are lactose intolerant to some extent. Lactose is the sugar in milk, and it is broken down in our intestines by the enzyme lactase. By the age of four, many of us have stopped producing that enzyme. The undigested lactose moves to the colon, where it ferments and causes bloating, gas, cramps, and sometimes diarrhea. The chances that you are lactose intolerant are particularly high if your ancestry is African American, Native American, Greek, Arab, Ashkenazi or Sephardic Jewish, or Oriental.

Another problem with large amounts of calcium from food is that calcium needs magnesium to be incorporated into your bones. If you do not have enough magnesium in your body to match the extra calcium from food, the excess calcium will collect in soft tissues instead of in bone and cause calcium deposits and arthritis.

Dairy products contain nine times as much calcium as magnesium. That means you need a lot of magnesium from some other source if you drink much milk or eat a lot of dairy products. This was no problem for our ancestors, before the arrival of dairy products. They had an abundant supply of magnesium for their modest calcium needs back then from the nuts, seeds, beans, and vegetables they ate. Their bodies had no need to evolve a magnesium-storing mechanism. But because their food was low in calcium, their bodies did evolve to store that mineral. As I've said in my book *Your Body Knows Best,* because of this storage mechanism, a little calcium goes a long way in our bodies.

Please don't misunderstand what I am saying! I am *not* saying that calcium is bad for you and doesn't help your bones. I'm saying that in order to have calcium build your bones, you must have enough magnesium to work with it. Magnesium helps calcium absorption and deposition in the bones, where it belongs. Calcium interferes with magnesium absorption. Magnesium decreases the demand for calcium. While we enrich our diet with calcium—we even add the mineral to orange juice and ingest a brand of antacids (Tums) for its calcium content—we eat a magnesium-impoverished diet. We eat less magnesium-rich food than our Stone Age ancestors did, such as leafy green vegetables, nuts, seeds, and sea vegetables. With the best intentions, we create a magnesium-calcium imbalance.

We even add to this imbalance by eating foods rich in sugar and by drinking alcohol, both of which increase magnesium excretion through the kidneys. We don't eat almonds because they contain too much fat. Almonds have a high magnesium content and would do much to help lay down calcium as bone. Chinese, Indian, and other Oriental foods are also high in magnesium. It's noteworthy that neither osteoporosis nor osteoarthritis is as great a health problem in the East as in the West.

I say all this even though I am fully aware that on August 13, 1997, the Institute of Medicine, a branch of the National Academy of Sciences, raised the recommended daily intake of calcium from 800 to 1000 milligrams for women in their thirties and forties, and from 800 to 1200 milligrams for women aged fifty and over. They also raised the RDAs for magnesium, phosphorus, vitamin D, and fluoride. I suggest that, unless you are monitoring your individual needs through tissue mineral analysis, you consider taking twice as much magnesium as calcium (taken as separate supplements at different times of the day) until you feel that a better balance between the two minerals has been achieved in your body. After that, taking the supplements in a 1:1 ratio probably makes good sense.

A magnesium deficiency can cause perimenopausal symptoms. Magnesium acts as a sedative within the body, and one of the most significant symptoms of a deficiency is a feeling of extreme edginess. Sudden sounds make you jump. Going easy on dairy products and avoiding foods artificially enriched with calcium should help. Taking a magnesium supplement of 500 to 1000 milligrams a day will build up your tissue level. But don't take a magnesium supplement after a meal, because the magnesium neutralizes stomach acids that you need for digestion. And don't forget that magnesium works with vitamin B_6 and zinc in very special ways to alleviate a broad spectrum of perimenopause symptoms.

Some Perimenopausal Symptoms Caused by Magnesium Deficiency

Nervousness
Anxiety
Irritability
Muscle tremors
Muscle cramps
Memory loss
Concentration problems

Apathy
Depression
Perspiration increase
Body odor increase
Urination increase
Constipation

Rejuvex

Many magnesium products are available on the market. The trick is to find one without added calcium. One such is Rejuvex. These nonprescription pills provide 125 percent of the Recommended Daily Allowance of magnesium, principally in the form of magnesium oxide. If your body level of magnesium is low, this easily obtained commercial product will help you rebuild the level and get rid of symptoms caused by magnesium deficiency.

The pills also contain, as principal ingredients, vitamins E, B_1, B_2, B_3, and B_6, thiamine, pantothenic acid, selenium, and manganese. Minor ingredients include dong quai, cellulose fiber, and raw glandular powders from bovine sources (mammary, ovary, uterus, adrenal, and pituitary).

The pills do not contain zinc. Taken with a zinc supplement, Rejuvex is a powerful remedy for many perimenopause symptoms. Follow the instructions on the label.

Tissue Mineral Analysis

Corinne's case history in this chapter shows the importance of using tissue mineral analysis of a hair sample to assess mineral levels in tissues that differ from those found in the blood. A hair sample reveals what has been going on in the body for three months, while blood constantly readapts to more immediate and short-term metabolic shifts. While I fully acknowledge that many practitioners dismiss hair analysis, I have consistently found it the missing link in subclinical assessment of mineral levels.

Hair analysis provides an accurate reflection of the body's mineral needs when you consider the following:

Hairs develop in skin follicles. As the hair cells grow in the follicle, they are exposed to blood, lymph, and extracellular fluids. Once the hair emerges from the follicle, its outer layers harden and thus lock in place the metabolic products that are present. This provides a lasting biological record of the metabolites that were present when the hair emerged.

To find out how to get a tissue mineral analysis of a hair sample, call Uni Key Health Systems at 1–800–888–4353. Uni Key does not do tissue mineral analysis directly, but can help connect you with a lab that does in association with my office.

Chapter 7

Natural Hormone Cream

Fighting Fatigue,
Listless Libido,
Irregular Periods,
and Osteoporosis

The Changing Diet helps stabilize your body's hormonal balance, and Peri Zappers #1 through #4 contribute vital nutrients that should make up for anything your body is missing in terms of nutrition. Many of my clients find that these remedies clear up their perimenopausal symptoms quite simply. But they are not enough for everyone. Now, if the Changing Diet and these Zapper nutrients don't prove powerful enough to alleviate your symptoms, my next recommendation is to use natural progesterone as a skin cream.

The Menstrual Cycle

To highlight the role of progesterone, let's review some familiar information about the menstrual cycle. Your cycle normally lasts twenty-six to twenty-eight days. The cycle begins with your brain sending a message to your ovaries to stimulate egg follicles. Only one egg fully ripens and moves, in its follicle, to the outer surface of the ovary. On ovulation, the follicle bursts, and the released egg travels down the fallopian tube to the uterus.

As the egg was ripening in the ovary, the lining of your uterus walls thickened and developed a network of blood veins. This was in expectation that the fertilized egg would become implanted on the lining and require nourishment. Only a fertilized egg becomes implanted. In the absence of a fertilized egg, the uterine lining is shed and menstruation begins. The cycle then begins again.

For a week or so after your period, estrogen is the dominant hormone. It stimulates the buildup of the uterine lining.

On approximately the twelfth day after your period began, your estrogen level peaks and begins to drop, just before you ovulate. After you ovulate, the empty follicle that held the egg starts to produce progesterone. The follicle is now called the corpus luteum (yellow body), and its progesterone is the dominant hormone of the second half of the menstrual cycle. Progesterone also stimulates the buildup of the uterine lining.

If the egg is not fertilized, both estrogen and progesterone levels drop sharply. If the egg is fertilized, the progesterone level remains high. Women in perimenopause quite often become pregnant, especially those who believe that they can't!

If you miss ovulation in a menstrual cycle, there is no empty follicle to become the corpus luteum. Therefore progesterone is not secreted by the ovary in sufficient quantities to counteract the effects of estrogen, and a hormonal imbalance—and symptoms—results. This condition is referred to as estrogen dominance. Dr. John R. Lee's pioneering work has helped us understand the varying effects of estrogen and progesterone as well as the characteristics of estrogen dominance.

Comparison of the Effects of
Estrogen and Progesterone

Estrogen	Progesterone
Stimulates uterine lining cell growth	Stabilizes uterine lining cell growth
Stimulates breast cell growth	Stabilizes breast cell growth
Adds to body fat	Helps burn body fat as fuel
Promotes water retention	Diuretic
Promotes depression	Antidepressant
Causes headaches	Does not cause headaches
Anti–thyroid hormone	Pro–thyroid hormone
Promotes blood clotting	Stabilizes blood clotting
Diminishes sex drive	Increases sex drive
Upsets blood sugar balance	Stabilizes blood sugar balance
Anti-zinc and pro-copper in body	Stabilizes zinc-copper balance in body
Lowers cell oxygen levels	Normalizes cell oxygen levels
Raises risk of uterine cancer	Prevents uterine cancer
Raises risk of breast cancer	Helps prevent breast cancer
Anti–bone building	Pro–bone building
Antivascular	Provascular

Characteristics of Estrogen Dominance

Bloating	Periods occasionally heavy
Breast swelling	Sex drive diminishment
Depression	Sugar cravings
Fat deposition on hips and thighs	Tiredness
Hypothyroid symptoms	Uterine fibroids
Mood swings	Water retention
Periods irregular	Weight gain

Benefits of Progesterone

Besides its ability to counteract the undesirable effects of estrogen, progesterone has been credited with fighting heart disease and cancer. In women in their thirties and forties, progesterone plays an active role in bone density; a high progesterone level is a major preventive against later osteoporosis.

After a fertilized egg settles on the uterus wall, ovarian progesterone cares for it. After the placenta develops, it, too, secretes progesterone. Progesterone levels continue high throughout pregnancy, which is why many women in the third trimester, and in spite of some physical discomfort, feel as good as they have ever felt in their lives. When her progesterone level falls sharply after the birth, the mother is apt to feel postpartum depression.

At menopause, the drop in progesterone level is twelve times greater than that in estrogen level (estrogen declines by 40 to 60 percent). Men have higher progesterone levels than some postmenopausal women.

By increasing body energy, probably by helping thyroid hormones work better, progesterone causes a very slight but often noticeable rise in your body temperature when you ovulate. This varies from woman to woman.

Jackie

Jackie, forty-four, came to my office asking for an energy-boosting diet. She complained of a total lack of energy, chronic tiredness, and constant fatigue. Her doctor had suspected hypothyroidism, but the results of her TSH and T4 blood tests indicated that her thyroid gland was functioning normally.

Jackie thought that maybe the kind of carbohydrate-loading diet used by athletes would give her more zest. I warned her that every blood sugar high on that kind of diet was followed by an even bigger low.

During our consultation, I soon found out that because of family tragedies, Jackie had undergone much stress in the past few years. In an almost accidental aside, she mentioned that she used estrogen patches. No, she hadn't filled that in on the form at the doctor's office as medication she was taking, because she had gotten the patches from a friend and didn't consider them medication.

As I saw it, she had become fatigued due to extended stress. Someone gave her the patches as a tonic. The estrogen interfered with the action of her thyroid hormones at the cell receptors. She developed hypothyroid symptoms, which she may have been predisposed to anyway, and these made it look like her thyroid was underfunctioning. I got her to throw out the patches and apply natural progesterone cream to her skin to rebuild her reserves. In three weeks, her major symptoms were gone. She still wasn't ready to run a mile, but now she had some energy. I suggested that she reduce the cream to minimal use, and, with the Changing Diet, supplements, and exercise, she soon became her take-charge self once again.

Natural Progesterone vs. Synthetic Progestin

As a natural substance, progesterone cannot be patented or trademarked or otherwise protected in the marketplace. It belongs to everyone. In order to make their commercial progesterone products exclusively owned brands, pharmaceutical companies deliberately alter the natural structure of the progesterone molecule and come up with a synthetic product called progestin. That strategy works well in the marketplace. The problem is that progestin works much less well than natural progesterone in your body.

The synthetically altered molecule is accepted by the progesterone receptors of your cells and passes on its message to the cell DNA. This message is never quite the same as that of natural progesterone. Your body does not feel completely right. You may notice that you are increasingly irritable, lose your temper more often, and feel at times emotionally unstable. Progestin, the synthetic form of progesterone, can intensify all your symptoms. Progestin does not match your body's chemistry exactly and can inhibit ovulation or suppress your body's own secretion of natural progesterone.

In the recent Postmenopausal Estrogen/Progestin Intervention Study (PEPI), researchers found that, for 875 healthy women, a combination of natural progesterone and estrogen more effectively minimized side effects—that is, symptoms—than a combination of progestin and estrogen.

There may be other consequences because of progesterone's role as a precursor of estrogen, testosterone, stress hormones, and other vital bodily substances. The fact that progesterone is a precursor of other substances is important. When a nonprecursor has fulfilled its functions in the body, it is broken down and excreted. Any potential for harmful effects goes with it. A precursor, on the other hand, can pass along to succeeding substances some of the harmful effects it possesses.

Either progestin won't work as a precursor or, worse still, it may produce an altered successor capable of all kinds of damage. These ill effects might not easily be traced to their source, or they might be subtle, manifesting themselves only over time.

Your body also has difficulty in breaking down progestin and excreting it. This creates a potential for toxic effects from unexcreted, partially broken down waste circulating in the system.

Concern about the potential harm of synthetic progestin is not widespread in the medical profession, and it receives little or no publicity compared with the full-page color ads from pharmaceutical companies. Dr. John R. Lee, a pioneer of women's health studies, is a noteworthy exception.

Dorothy

"I was the bad girl in convent school," Dorothy told me. "We had to wear a school uniform. When we got out of school, I always hiked mine up so it was a miniskirt. I can't remember a time back then when I wasn't boy crazy." She sighed at the memory and added bitterly, "Look at me now."

With her pert nose, blue eyes, wavy golden hair, and a generous, often smiling, mouth, Dorothy, a part-time bank employee, was an attractive, instantly likable person. At forty-three, she was tiny and bouncy, but her state of mind was not as sunny as her appearance led people to believe.

"I know my husband must be running around—probably nothing serious so far," she said. "He's having a lot of late evenings at work. I know that everyone has to work harder just to stay in place nowadays. But I know that's not why he stays out. He's got a better reason. He's not getting any loving at home, so he's finding it elsewhere."

As we talked, I couldn't help noticing that Dorothy felt more comfortable talking about her lack of sex drive from her husband's point of view than from her own. I mentioned this to her.

She nodded. "I've been listening to his complaints long enough. For once, the man is more verbal. I don't know how to answer. I was always a sex kitten. I don't know why I'm now an ice princess."

Dorothy had been to a doctor and had a blood test of her hormone levels. Her estrogen level had come back normal, as had some other levels whose names she couldn't recall (probably FSH and LH). From her test result, the doctor assured her that she didn't have a hormone problem. Nor did she have any sign of a medical disorder. The doctor concluded that her loss of interest in sex was probably due to an emotional or psychological problem.

"I wasn't going to see a shrink," Dorothy said forcefully, her eyes blazing even now at the thought. "I told the doctor I wasn't crazy. She said you don't have to be crazy and that I had a misunderstanding of psychological therapy. I said that although I couldn't explain why I didn't want sex anymore, I was certain it was for a *physical* reason. The thought of sex didn't repulse me, like it might for a psychological reason. I explained that I just don't care. I'm indifferent. Not me really—*my body* is indifferent."

Dorothy was a bit surprised, I think, when I dropped the subject of sex and started asking her about apparently unrelated symptoms. No, she didn't have weight gain. She wasn't particularly irritable or nervous. In fact, just the opposite. She felt sluggish, especially in the mornings. No headaches. Food cravings? Don't even mention the words. In the last couple of years, she had become a coffee and pastry addict. She found that they helped her get going in the morning. A large café latte and a blueberry or cherry sweet roll helped her through her afternoon sinking spell. And she often had coffee and apple pie with women friends when her husband had to "work" late.

I asked if her periods were regular.

"For the past three years or so, I've had several very light ones in a row, followed by a heavy one, and then more light ones," she said. "But I've never missed a period."

It was clear that this information seemed unimportant to her. Yet all the pieces of the puzzle were there; she just didn't see how they connected. But her instincts were good, as they are in many women. She had instinctively felt that her body was more a cause of her troubles than her mind. I told her that in this she was almost certainly correct.

Although Dorothy didn't have some of the more typical symptoms of estrogen dominance, such as weight gain (particularly around the abdomen, hips, and thighs), water retention, irritability, and depression, she had one of the most important classic signs—decreased sex drive. This was probably caused by her not ovulating and consequently lacking corpus luteum secretion of progesterone. The resulting estrogen dominance was responsible for her loss of sex drive, or libido.

After telling her that she first would have to break her caffeine and high-sugar pastry habits, I put her on the Changing Diet. In addition to that, I recommended natural progesterone cream for her to rub on her skin in order to build up and stabilize her tissue level of progesterone. The higher level of progesterone would counteract the libido-diminishing effects of estrogen.

Dorothy spent some months falling off the caffeine and sugar wagon, and she couldn't really stay on the Changing Diet until she had broken those habits. During those months, however, she faithfully used the natural progesterone cream on her skin as recommended. Gradually, she began to feel a bit more frisky in the bedroom. Last I heard, she was on the diet and feeling quite her kittenish self again. And things seemed to have improved at her husband's workplace; he didn't have to put in all those evening hours anymore.

Purchasing and Applying a Cream

You need to be selective when buying a cream, because some creams contain only a tiny percentage of progesterone or none at all. Some creams use extracts from soybeans (which are also used for phytoestrogens), and others are based on the wild yam (*Dioscorea*). Diosgenin is the yam's active ingredient. Although a

★ *Ann Louise's* ★
All-Star Peri Zapper #5

Natural Progesterone Cream

Progesterone cream balances estrogen dominance symptoms, such as decreased sex drive, depression, abnormal
blood sugar levels, fatigue, fuzzy thinking, irritability, thyroid dysfunction, water retention, bone loss, fat gain, and
low adrenal function.

Massage a high-quality progesterone cream into the
soft, capillary-rich skin of your face, neck, upper chest,
breasts, inner arms, palms and backs of hands, and soles.
Rotate skin areas daily so that you don't saturate the subdermal receptors. Apply from the twelfth to twenty-sixth
day of your menstrual cycle. Use a total of 1/8 to 1/4 teaspoon daily to start, in one or two applications a day.

---

number of creams make claims for it, research has shown that
diosgenin *in natural plant form* does not bind with human cell
progesterone receptors, meaning that these creams are useless as
progesterone sources.

Diosgenin has to be processed in a lab into progesterone.
Some of the creams that contain diosgenin from wild yams also
contain lab-grade progesterone, and some do not. Investigators
have shown that creams containing only wild yam extract do not
significantly boost a woman's progesterone level. They have also
shown that creams that contain lab-grade progesterone do boost
the body's progesterone level.

So, the word *natural* when applied to progesterone doesn't
mean exactly what it usually means. Here the term *natural* means
that the plant progesterone molecule is identical to the human
progesterone molecule, distinguishing it from the pharmaceutical
progestin, whose molecule is slightly different from human pro-

gesterone. Thus, both natural progesterone and deliberately altered progestin are derived from either wild yam or soybean and are processed in the laboratory.

Hair Loss and Skipped Periods

If you have hair loss and skipped periods, they may be connected. Lack of ovulation in a skipped period can cause the adrenal cortex to secrete the steroid hormone androstenedione as an alternative chemical precursor for the manufacture of other hormones. This steroid hormone is associated with some male characteristics, one of which is male pattern baldness. But when you raise your progesterone level with natural progesterone cream, your androstenedione level will gradually decline and your hair will grow back normally. Be patient—hair growth is slow and it may take several months before you notice a difference.

According to Dr. John R. Lee, in a normal menstrual cycle your body produces 20 to 24 milligrams of progesterone a day for twelve to fourteen days. This comes to a total of approximately 250 milligrams of progesterone for each menstrual cycle. A two-ounce tube or jar of 1.6 percent (by weight) or 3 percent (by volume) cream contains about 950 milligrams of progesterone. Half of such a tube or jar, applied externally, should provide more than enough progesterone for one menstrual cycle. Apply a total 1/8 to 1/4 teaspoon of cream daily. After a week or more, apply a total of up to 1/2 teaspoon cream daily if your symptoms require it. You may apply the cream as often as you like, so long as you don't exceed the daily total. To avoid saturating the receptors beneath your skin in any one area, apply the cream to different areas each day. Soft skin rich in capillaries is the most suitable, such as that found in the neck, upper chest, breasts, inner arms, palms, backs of hands, and soles.

The progesterone from skin cream is absorbed transdermally into the fatty layer beneath your skin. You will probably notice your skin becoming more resilient and moist in the areas where you often apply the cream. The progesterone is taken from the fatty layer beneath your skin by the bloodstream, which distributes it throughout your system. This is not an overnight effect. It may even take several weeks, or occasionally a couple of months, for the progesterone level to build in tissues and make its effects felt. But don't try to rush the process by taking bigger doses. Too much of any hormone at one time can have the opposite effect of the one desired.

The natural progesterone cream that I recommend most is Pro-Gest, from Professional & Technical Services. You should be able to find it in health food stores. Or you can order it by mail from Uni Key Health Systems at 1–800–888–4353.

Oral capsules of natural progesterone are also available. The progesterone is in micronized form, which ensures that it will not be largely lost when processed by the liver.

Creams with More Than 400 Milligrams of Natural Progesterone per Ounce

Angel Care, from Angel Care

Bio Balance, from Garon Pharmaceuticals

Equilibrium, from Equilibrium Lab

Femme Naturale, from Sarati International

NatraGest, from Broadmoore Labs

OstaDerm, from Bezwecken

PhytoGest, from Karuna Corp.

Pro-Alo, from HealthWatchers

ProBalance, from Springboard

Pro-G, from TriMedica

Pro-Gest, from Professional & Technical Services

Progonal, from Bezwecken

Chapter 8

Making Exercise More Fun

hen your blood sugar becomes stable on the Changing Diet, your blood level of the hormone glucagon becomes elevated. Whereas insulin adds to body fat, glucagon helps burn it away as fuel for energy. The great thing about having a high glucagon level is that it means you are burning body fat even when you are not physically active—even while you sit here reading this page, even while you sleep in bed!

- Body Fat
- Fuel
- Energy
- Activity

Obviously, you burn off much more body fat if you are active. You use up more body fat as fuel, measured in calories, as your metabolic rate increases. This has been known for many years, and most traditional diets are based on this concept alone. The new generation of diets that take the body's hormones into consideration has completely transformed progressive and informed dieting. Nutrients evoke hormonal responses from the body, and the hormones then control how the nutrients are put to use in the body.

It's now recognized widely that exercise also evokes hormonal responses from the body. Aerobic exercise reduces your insulin level and elevates your glucagon level. Anaerobic exercise, such as strength training, causes the body to secrete human growth hormone. This hormone, a builder and repairer of muscle tissue in adults, is the great white shark of fat burners. Glucagon promotes vasodilation, the expansion of blood vessels, so that more nutrient- and oxygen-bearing blood can reach muscle tissues and bear away lactic acid when leaving. But fat-burning hormones are not the only ones that respond to exercise. In fact, exercise is one of the healthiest, most effective, and most natural ways to combat depression or stress. This is because exercise releases endorphins, neurotransmitters that heighten mood.

For many years, I have noticed how exercise helps just about every symptom for perimenopause. Although I'm not certain how this exactly works, we certainly do know that exercise helps weight control, manages stress, and lessens the risk of osteoporosis and heart disease. I can make an educated guess that exercise also enables your metabolism to work better and more intensely, so that you get more benefit from whatever nutrients your body is processing. Healing oils, vitamins, minerals—they all seem to be more intensely absorbed by the body when you exercise regularly. This means that symptoms are alleviated or disappear faster.

When your body is reasonably fit, most of your bodily systems are in fairly good balance. When only your hormones are out of balance and the rest of your body is more or less in balance, the Zapper nutrients are free to work on your hormone problem. But if your bodily systems are sluggish and you are out of condition due to a sedentary life, those Zapper nutrients will probably be utilized somewhere else in your system before they ever reach your hormones!

Lightening Up on Exercise

Twenty years ago, we were being told that to gain any health benefits from exercise, it had to be incredibly strenuous. No pain, no gain. Most people had sense enough to ignore this over-the-top advice and go on with whatever felt good for their bodies, even if this did not conform to the expectations of the American College of Sports Medicine and similar institutions. Nowadays, people are being encouraged to do five minutes of gardening, fifteen minutes of walking to the store, pushing a stroller, playing with a dog, raking leaves. It all adds up. You burn the same amount of calories walking briskly that you do running.

"Some women who exercise strenuously stop menstruating because of low body-fat levels," Dr. Mona M. Shangold, director of the Center for Women's Health and Sports Gynecology in Philadelphia, told the *New York Times*. She added that cessation of menses (amenorrhea) can strike any woman of child-bearing age but most frequently occurs among teenagers and younger women.

Much of the really worrisome overexercising that I have seen involves young girls being encouraged by their parents to excel at sports. What makes it heartbreaking is that the young girls usually do it out of fear of disappointing their over-zealous parents. But some women in their thirties and forties also suffer from too much physical activity, far more often than you might imagine. However, their activity is rarely sports related. Cheryl comes to mind.

Cheryl

Cheryl, at thirty-eight, had two teenaged kids and a husband who had trouble holding down a job. She herself worked full-time at her job of nine years, and in addition she drove the kids to practices and appointments, helped them with schoolwork, cooked, cleaned, did yardwork, and regularly checked on her husband's widowed mother, who had diabetes and lived alone. Her husband spent a lot of time away from the house, "looking for work" usually getting home for dinner and then flopping into an easy chair. Cheryl felt constantly fatigued and thought I should put her on a special diet.

"What you need," I offered, "may not be a nutritionist but more moderation in your life. Perhaps your husband could pitch in more."

She immediately started defending her husband, saying what a special kind of person he was and how hard he found it to adapt and so forth. While she was talking, she got out of her chair and started tidying up my office. I was preparing for a speaking engagement, and I had arranged papers on the floor. Cheryl picked them all up, placed them neatly on shelves, and sat down again, all the while talking to me. I looked at her and realized that she was not conscious of what she had just done.

Even before discussing her other symptoms or testing her for clinical deficiencies, it was obvious to me that her overriding problem was one of overdoing. She was an overachiever, trying to be a superwoman. With no help from her husband, she was overextending herself. I told her so, and she walked out of my office. I never saw her again.

Housework is exercise. Housework very often is *strenuous* exercise. Taking care of young children is always strenuous exercise. You'd be surprised how many women worry about not having energy enough to go jogging after a day packed with more physical activity than most professional athletes have.

Vigorous Walking

Moderate exercise has been shown to help all our bodily systems. Walking a mile a day has been found to reduce women's risk of losing bone density as they get older. A minimum of four hours of exercise a week reduces the risk of getting breast cancer by 37 percent, researchers found in a recent study of 25,000 Norwegian women. The CDC calculated that a sedentary lifestyle is a contributing cause to about a quarter million deaths every year in the

United States. In 1991 a British Heart Foundation Report implied that lack of exercise was a health risk equivalent to smoking a pack of cigarettes a day.

Brisk, vigorous walking is the most convenient form of exercise for most of us.

For walking to qualify as beneficial exercise, it must be vigorous, so make sure to move your arms. In hot weather, you can walk early in the morning or after sundown. In cold weather, bundle up or get on a treadmill or Nordic Track.™

If you walk vigorously for thirty minutes or so five days a week, I guarantee you will *feel* better and *look* better in a matter of a few weeks.

Walking your way to feeling and looking better is simple. You don't need special equipment, just a comfortable pair of shoes. You can walk alone or with friends. You can vary your route so you don't get bored. As you walk, you can pray, meditate, or plot. You can listen to music (no cellular phone please except as an emergency or safety measure). So if walking is so easy, what's stopping us? Why don't more women walk?

Because we haven't got time. Ask anyone. There's really only one answer to that objection. You have to make time. You do that by examining the structure of your days, finding that half hour somewhere, and then treating it as seriously as you do your other duties and appointments. Apart from personal and family responsibilities and your job, how many other activities of your day are as

Ann Louise's All-Star Peri Zapper #6

Exercise

Be vigorously active for a half hour five days a week. Do housework, garden, walk briskly, cycle, swim, dance, have fun. Do different things each day—and do what you enjoy.

important as getting rid of perimenopause symptoms? Exercise will really help you do that, if you give it a chance.

Janice

A sedentary occupation and a fondness for soft drinks are dual problems for American women of all ages. It takes a lot of exercise to beat that combination. But every bit of exercise amounts to a fraction of a pound of body fat not put on. Every bit helps. So I told Janice.

It did no good. So far as I could estimate, Janice drank three to four liters of Coca-Cola a day. At her job as a telemarketer, where she often put in twelve-hour days, she ate anything that happened to be around, such as pizza slices, candy bars, doughnuts, or even someone's salad if they didn't want it. She apparently never actually purchased food. And of course she never had any exercise. At forty-one, she lived at her own apartment sometimes and stayed with her seventy-something mother and her boyfriend, both of whom lived near her, at other times. The only things that weren't vague in Janice's life, so far as I could see, were her perimenopausal symptoms.

Her migraines were totally debilitating, sometimes lasting for days, during which she would lie in bed in a darkened room, trying various over-the-counter remedies in what sounded to me like dangerous amounts. They didn't provide her lasting relief, but she tried them over and over again. Insomnia, fatigue, and occasional crawling skin sensations rounded out the picture. Nothing that I recommended seemed to help, either—if, that is, she really followed the advice, which I never knew.

Then Janice got downsized, in both senses of the word. Out of her present job and interviewing for another, she discovered how her weight and appearance were stumbling blocks for employment. She came to see me now on a weekly basis, and I was amazed each week to see the improvement in her. Having lost about fifteen pounds in two months, she had started cooking for herself and buying new clothes. I figured that she was walking about two hours a day and drinking one liter of Coke.

"Don't go back to telemarketing," I pleaded.

"I thought I might get a job as a bookkeeper or secretary," Janice said.

I shook my head. There had to be something else, something active. There was. She now delivers and installs office telephone and computer network systems. On her feet all day, she must be fifty pounds lighter than a couple of years ago. She's on the Changing Diet and M 'n' M supplements, and except for an occasional headache that passes within a few hours, her perimenopause symptoms have disappeared. Before she started getting exercise, neither diet nor supplements had brought her any relief. I suspect that this was because her blood sugar was so unstable—she may have been on the verge of adult-onset diabetes—that her system was not metabolizing nutrients very well. Exercise got it going again.

Exercises to Prevent Osteoporosis

Do keep in mind that some kind of resistance or weight-bearing exercise is needed to prevent osteoporosis. Walking, running, bicycling, aerobics, light weight-lifting or any other form of exercise that makes a lot of use of the legs and hips is needed. Twenty minutes to an hour three times a week is adequate. Research has shown that women who did this kind of exercise for an hour three times a week increased their bone density by 2.6 percent in one year.

No matter what exercise program you decide to follow, the key is to . . . keep moving!

Chapter 9

Taking the Distress Out of Stress

*A*re your nerves frazzled over family and work, and is your dress size on the rise again? Most of us in our thirties and forties are under a great deal of stress trying to juggle family and career. Many of us find it increasingly hard not to put on extra pounds, let alone lose any weight. Two sets of hormones are already involved here: stress hormones and blood sugar hormones. So when our ovarian hormones start acting up at the same time, it would be nice to find a magic pill that could restore better balance to all three of these hormone systems. Such a magic pill exists, but it's not manufactured by a big pharmaceutical company or a cutting-edge biotech firm. You handle it every day. It's called food, and its nutrients can restore balance to all three hormone systems. Add a little exercise for spice.

No hormonal makeover can be complete, however, without some work on your stress hormones. Stress amplifies or magnifies our perimenopausal symptoms. Frequently, when we get stress under control, our symptoms fade or completely disappear, even symptoms that aren't apparently connected to stress. How do we deal with stress? In two ways. First we understand it, and then we manage it. We break stress down into its component parts, making it easier to handle. Then we look at what really gets to us and what doesn't and learn how to manage the really annoying things and avoid a cumulative buildup of distress.

Breathing, meditation, and enjoyable exercise are popular and effective ways of managing the unavoidable stress of modern life. The nutritional approach is less well known, and it is the one we will discuss here. In this approach, you take nutrients designed to restore your adrenal glands, the glands that secrete your stress hormones. These nutrients are not meant to replace exercise, meditation, and other relaxation techniques but to reinforce them.

Stress as a Three-Step Process

Almost every day in the media, we are told that technology and modern life are killing us. We are warned about stress and what it can do to us. We are given advice, most of it from people who obviously have never had to work and raise a family at the same time. Each of us has her own private solutions. We say to ourselves that we would have less stress if we had a more romantic husband or more obedient children or longer vacations. In seeking individual solutions, we are using our common sense, because we recognize that stress must be dealt with on an individual basis.

A question that has intrigued the experts is why something is stressful to some people but not to others. Researchers Richard S. Lazarus and Susan Folkman, in working with the stress caused by anxiety, showed how some people *perceive* a thing as threatening while others don't. Those who perceive danger become anxious and stressful, while the others don't. Whether or not what you percieve is actually dangerous is irrelevant; the fact that you perceive it as threatening is what counts.

A federal panel of medical researchers decided that the word *stress* itself was too vague. They recommended that the following terms be used. We call the thing that we perceive as threatening a *stressor*. The stressor causes an unpleasant emotional, psychological, or physical sensation in us, which we call *distress*. The distress that we feel may or may not have a *consequence*. As an example, suppose you suddenly wondered whether you had turned off the stove before leaving the house. That thought—it doesn't have to be something physical—is the stressor. It causes you distress, in this case in the form of anxiety. You may shrug off this worry, in which case there will be no consequence. Or you may run a series of worst-case scenarios through your mind, like your house burning down. In that case, the consequence of your distress (anxiety) may be a fluttering heart and shortness of breath.

- Stressor
- Distress
- Consequence

At first, this formula may not seem useful. But think of something in your life that you find very stressful. Think of the stressor and why you perceive it as such. Consider the sensations of distress it arouses in you. And, finally, what consequences or symptoms does the distress cause in you? If you can make a change in any of those three steps in the stress process, you can interrupt the process and prevent your body from experiencing distress.

An interesting change has come about in the way that experts look at stressors. For years, stressors were evaluated according to their power to cause distress. There is even a chart ranking stressors, with "death of a spouse" ranked at the top. But clinicians pointed out that, first of all, such major stressful events are rare in most people's lives and, second, most people handle such major stressors very well. What causes distress in everyday life, the clinicians said, is the cumulative effect of daily hassles, all the minor stressful events during the day, such as getting stuck in traffic or not being able to find a phone number. All these little wisps of stress gather into a dark cloud.

The third step of the stress process is of special significance to women with perimenopausal symptoms. Distress has consequences in your body. In general, you may be more prone to react to stress with an intensifying of symptoms you already have from other causes. If you already suffer from, say, fatigue, sleeplessness, or irritability, stress can give these symptoms new life, as I'm sure you already know. But the consequences are not limited to perimenopausal symptoms. For instance, a stressor that causes a healthy woman to have a rapidly beating heart could cause a woman with a heart condition to develop further complications. If you already have perimenopause symptoms, you don't need the consequences of stress added to them!

Hormones and Stress

When you perceive a stressor, hormones from your brain pass through your bloodstream and alert your adrenal glands, which are located over your kidneys. In response, the cortex of each adrenal gland secretes corticosteroid hormones, one of which is cortisol. The amount of cortisol in the blood increases twentyfold

Ann Louise's
All-Star Peri Zapper #7

Destressing Stress

Remember that you perceive a stressor as such and that stress is a three-step process:
- Stressor
- Distress
- Consequence

The process can be interrupted at any step.

in response to stressors. This hormone permits the body to vastly speed up its blood-sugar-burning capacity to provide an instant surge of energy. Cortisol also assists in the release of amino acids to repair damaged tissue.

The corticosteroid hormones cause your heart to beat faster in response to a stressor, in order to pump oxygen-bearing blood more quickly to your tissues. They make you breathe more rapidly, to provide more oxygen to the blood. And they have a feedback system to the brain that permits them to intensify or ease up in secretion according to what you are presently perceiving.

Too much of a stress hormone from the brain in the bloodstream can lead to diabetes or high blood pressure. Problems with the hormone feedback system can cause chronic anxiety or depression. The involvement of corticosteroid hormones with perimenopausal symptoms is complex. It is rarely possible to know whether these hormones initiate a symptom or simply aggravate one that is already present.

The interaction of corticosteroid hormones with the sympathetic and parasympathetic nervous systems is a delicate balancing act. This interaction controls all the bodily systems not under direct control of the brain, such as breathing, heartbeat, and intestinal movements. So when something stressful knocks the wind out of you, makes your heart stand still, or twists your stomach in a knot, this is close to what is actually happening. While it may be unpleasant to experience, this physical reaction enables you to respond in an emergency.

Now enter technology and the modern world. Our bodily systems have evolved to respond to emergencies, such as the sudden appearance of a mammoth or saber-toothed tiger from behind a rock, but urban life in developed countries presents us instead with a nonstop stream of minor emergencies (hassles) at a frequency that neither our minds nor bodies have adapted to. The result can be that the adrenal glands enter a mode of almost constantly secreting small amounts of corticosteroid hormones into the bloodstream. With constant daily hassles over time, the adrenal cortex system can become less sensitive and wear out.

Nutrients for the Adrenal Glands

Regardless of whether your stress is physical or mental in origin, the corticosteroid hormones are those that enable your body to respond. The cortex of your adrenal glands is kept busy during stressful periods. The best way to look after the health of this gland and to refresh it during and after stressful periods is to ingest nutrients known to supply its needs. And since the hormone progesterone is the precursor to the corticosteroid hormones, its continued use will benefit the adrenals as well.

Sea vegetables, available in dried form at most health food stores, are rich in minerals and restore many of the minerals used up during stressful periods, such as magnesium, potassium, phosphorus, and iodine. The trace minerals zinc, selenium, manganese, and chromium are also found in sea vegetables. Sea vegetables can be eaten either as a side dish or as a condiment.

Green vegetables (broccoli, collards, kale, mustard greens), yellow-orange vegetables (carrots, squash, pumpkin, sweet potatoes), and fruit (bananas, cantaloupe, strawberries) are rich in many minerals consumed in stressful periods. Yes, I know that some of these are less than desirable on the glycemic index, so eat them with some quality protein and healthy fat when possible to balance blood sugar levels. You can get iron from legumes and zinc and manganese from eggs and meat. You may feel a craving for chocolate when under stress. Chocolate has some of the minerals you require (especially magnesium), but its high sugar content makes it one of the least desirable sources.

B-complex vitamins are often called "antistress vitamins" because of their calming effects. B_2 is particularly vital to the adrenal glands, as is pantothenic acid. Legumes, desiccated liver, and whole grains are recommended food sources. Blackstrap molasses (high in sugar) and brewer's yeast (a yeast promoter) are less desirable.

The need for vitamin C skyrockets during periods of great stress. Up to 3000 milligrams a day can be taken during such periods, and even higher amounts (5000 to 10,000 milligrams) during times of allergy, colds, or flu. The body can make better use of the high dose if it is divided into several smaller doses taken over the course of the day. For general perimenopause needs, I recommend 500 milligrams of vitamin C every three hours. Citrus fruits, cantaloupe, broccoli, green peppers, and rose hips are good food sources of vitamin C.

Zinc and manganese are especially needed by the adrenal glands during periods of high stress. Both zinc and manganese are found in pumpkin seeds, nuts, eggs, and lean beef. Sea vegetables are also good sources of trace minerals zinc and manganese.

I have found the Uni Key Adrenal Formula to be the most supportive for my clients' adrenal glands. Uni Key Adrenal Formula, from Uni Key (1–800–888–4353), consists of caplets, each containing vitamins A, B_5, B_6, and C, zinc, tyrosine, and freeze-dried raw bovine adrenal, adrenal cortex, spleen, and liver. These glandular extracts are tissue concentrates from animal glands and organs. Research has shown that these animal extracts carry the DNA/RNA blueprint of the gland or organ into the body because they are organ-specific.

Ann Louise's All-Star Peri Zapper #8

Adrenal Refresher

At times of a lot of stress, replacing lost minerals and vitamins can help the adrenal glands secrete stress hormones. Try the following:

- B complex vitamins
- Vitamin C, 500 milligrams every three hours
- Adrenal gland extract
- Green and yellow-orange vegetables
- Sea vegetables as a condiment

Exercise, relaxation techniques, meditation, and breathing techniques ease stress, too. So does talking over your problems with a friend. One thing may work best one day, and something else the next.

DHEA and Pregnenolone

The adrenal cortex makes small amounts of all the sex hormones but makes large amounts of dehydroepiandrosterone (DHEA) in both men and women. The role of DHEA is not fully understood. There's no doubt, however, that it is intimately tied to the metabolic processes that yield progesterone, estrogen, testosterone, and the stress hormone cortisol. Cholesterol is the originating molecule for all these compounds, including pregnenolone (the grandmother of corticosteroid hormones) and DHEA (the mother of corticosteroid hormones). Taking nonprescription doses of DHEA or pregnenolone is claimed to confer all kinds of health benefits on users, including protection against aging, burning muscle pain, depression, fatigue, stress, diabetes, lupus, and cancer.

The problem with taking DHEA and pregnenolone is that they are hormones involved in little-known biochemical interactions, which means that each has a wealth of potential side effects. The side effects that may be associated with long-term use of DHEA or pregnenolone are simply not known. There have already been complaints from women taking DHEA of growth of facial hair and deepening of the voice. But the most serious potential side effect is the stimulation of breast cancer, because DHEA can raise estrogen levels. Many perimenopausal women are too estrogen-dominant to begin with, as I have pointed out time and again.

According to biochemist William C. Fioretti of Mannatech, Inc., in Coppell, Texas, certain wild yam extracts that contain the diosgenin steroid can be converted into DHEA in the laboratory through a series of up to eight chemical reactions. The Mannatech product Plus (which contains wild yam and synergistic nutrients) has been monitored by a number of health care practitioners, who found that it raises DHEA levels in some cases.

My suggestion is that, instead of taking possibly dangerous hormones, you should boost the adrenal glands, which secrete these hormones, with adrenal glandulars or the Plus product. However, if you are still considering taking straight DHEA, have the following blood tests at your doctor's: DHEA, DHEAS, and serum and free testosterone and estradiol. In this way, you and your physician can monitor your baseline levels and retest to adjust dosage at regular intervals. A state-of-the-art twenty-four-hour urine test is now available for DHEA and its metabolites. (See Resources section.)

Hypothyroidism

The connection between the thyroid gland in the throat and the menstrual cycle was first noted by physicians a hundred years ago, after women who had had their thyroid removed developed menstrual irregularities. In the years that followed, the positive effects of thyroid therapy on menstrual disorders, infertility, miscarriages, depression, diminished sex drive, and perimenopause gradually became recognized—only to be forgotten again.

Dr. John R. Lee has observed that many perimenopausal women exhibit symptoms of hypothyroidism (underperformance of the thyroid gland) even with normal thyroid levels. He has theorized that estrogen excess and progesterone deficiency may be the cause. Raising progesterone levels through use of natural progesterone cream or supplements often normalizes thyroid activity without medication.

Dr. Broda O. Barnes developed the Barnes basal temperature test as an indicator of possible thyroid deficiency. In use since the early 1940s in various forms, this test is simple, and you can do it at home. After you have been using natural progesterone for several months, to see if you still may be suffering from hypothyroidism—rather than an estrogen-induced thyroid dysfunction that mimicks underperformance of the thyroid gland—do the following for at least one week, recording the average temperature—you should avoid days ten–fourteen of your cycle as your temperature may be elevated because of ovulation:

○ Shake a thermometer down as far as it will go, and place it next to your bed before going to sleep.

○ When you wake in the morning, before getting out of bed, without any mental or physical activity, place the thermometer under your armpit.

○ Lie quietly for ten minutes, and then read the thermometer.

The following readings are indicative of thyroid states:

97.8–98.2   Normally functioning thyroid

Above 98.2   Hyperthyroid or possible infection

Below 97.8   Possible hypothyroid

Dr. Barnes recommended natural thyroid preparations. Today cyclic naturally time-released thyroid therapy preparations are available through compounding pharmacies. (See Resources section.)

Some nutrients are specifically thyroid-friendly, and a deficiency in any one of them may result in thyroid dysfunction. The important thyroid supporting nutrients include the following with a suggested dosage most commonly recommended by nutritional experts:

Nutrient	Dosage
Vitamin B_2	15 milligrams
Vitamin B_6	25 to 50 milligrams
Vitamin A	25,000 international units
Vitamin E	400 international units
Zinc	20 to 30 milligrams
Iron	10 to 15 milligrams
Selenium	100 to 200 micrograms

| Iodine | 50 to 150 micrograms |
| Tyrosine | 250 milligrams |

Foods that may interfere with thyroid function when consumed excessively include cauliflower, cabbage, broccoli, brussels sprouts, and soy products.

Chapter 10

Estrogen and Phytoestrogens

*Zapping Hot Flashes,
Night Sweats, and Depression*

Many women suffer severe perimenopause symptoms for years. Many suffer the symptoms untreated, and many others treat hormonal symptoms with drugs like Prozac, sleeping pills, and mood elevators. We do have another choice, however, and that's what this book is about. For much of perimenopause, nutrient deficiencies, a low level of progesterone, and exhausted adrenal glands are frequent causes of hormonal imbalance and consequent symptoms. As we approach menopause, however, our estrogen level may start to fluctuate. Hot flashes are an almost certain indicator of this.

We can take mild plant estrogens—phytoestrogens—to alleviate our symptoms without condemning ourselves to a regimen of unpleasant synthetic hormones for the rest of our lives. Phytoestrogens are found in plant foods such as soybeans and in herbs such as dong quai and black cohosh. According to Dr. Christiane Northrup, these plant estrogens perform a balancing act by smoothing fluctuating hormone levels. Phytoestrogens respond to your body's individual needs by stimulating estrogen (and progesterone) production if levels are low, and lowering hormone levels that are too high. Before looking at this option, we need to take a look at the hormone estrogen itself. I particularly want to emphasize how little we know about this hormone, a drawback that is rarely acknowledged in the many references to it in the media.

About Estrogen

Most of us have heard both that estrogen improves the health of the heart, blood vessels, bones, brain, uterus, and breasts and that it is implicated in breast cancer, uterine cancer, ovarian cancer, autoimmune diseases, fibroids, asthma, mood swings, and migraines. Researchers find it hard to say where the boundaries of estrogen's powers lie or to untangle single estrogen threads from the whole estrogen tapestry. Moreover, they have had to change much of their previous thinking about this hormone because of some unexpected discoveries about how estrogen actually controls target cells.

Hormones like estrogen bind with cell receptors to form molecules that go directly to the cell's DNA to issue instructions. It was always assumed that this was a simple on-off process, like a light switch. The process was off when the receptor was empty, and on when the hormone filled its receptor. But our bodies are more complicated than that.

Benita Katzenellenbogen and co-workers at the University of Illinois found that different kinds of estrogen and estrogenlike drugs, on settling into a receptor, caused the resulting molecule to assume different shapes. The shape of the combined estrogen receptor molecule affected the choice of DNA genes that received instructions. For example, one shape might affect bone genes but not breast genes.

Difference in molecule shape may account for some of the distinct effects produced by different kinds of both natural estrogen and artificial estrogen. But researchers saw its immediate applicability to estrogenlike drugs. Molecule shape could refine the sledgehammer effect of estrogenlike drugs such as tamoxifen. Tamoxifen blocks estrogen's stimulation of cell growth in the breast and thereby helps prevent a recurrence of breast cancer. But, at the same time, the drug stimulates growth in other tissues. In bone, this is welcome. In the uterus, where tamoxifen stimulates the growth of lining cells, it can lead to uterine cancer.

One estrogenlike drug in the final stages of clinical testing avoids such broad effects. Eli Lilly's Raloxifene is an osteoporosis preventive that also protects the heart but does not stimulate cell proliferation in the uterus and breast. Glaxo Wellcome has a similar drug, soon to be tested, that presently bears the catchy name of GW5638.

Bert W. O'Malley, chairperson of the cell biology department at Baylor College of Medicine in Houston, told the *New York Times* that estrogen-receptor molecule shape is only part of the story. Mother Nature had another trick up her sleeve. When the estrogen-receptor molecule arrives at the DNA to deliver its message, two kinds of proteins are drawn to the site, coactivators and corepressors. If coactivators are in the majority, the hormone's message is passed on to the genes. However, if corepressors are in the majority, the message may be passed on in a weakened form or not at all.

"The cell doesn't necessarily want genes to be turned on all the time," Dr. O'Malley said, "so it has both an accelerator and a brake, just like a car."

Dr. O'Malley and colleagues showed that tamoxifen, for example, can be changed from an antiestrogen to an estrogen by changing the levels of coactivators and corepressors. Additionally, the levels of coactivators and corepressors in any particular tissue vary from woman to woman. Thus tamoxifen could work one way in one woman and another way in another woman.

"You can give a hundred women the same amount of hormone," O'Malley told the *Times* reporter, "and the dose will turn out to be too much for some women and not enough for others. In the future, we should be able to measure the sensitivity to a particular hormone in a given tissue and predict the ideal dose for each woman."

In a further twist, it is known that the sensitivity of a woman's tissues can change over time.

Even as researchers were digesting all this new information, they found that estrogen had been concealing a big secret from them. Estrogen had another receptor! All along, medical investigators had assumed that they were dealing with just one. Now they called the receptor they had known about the alpha receptor, and the second one the beta receptor. The beta receptor proved to be present in organs that had not been thought to be under the influence of estrogen, such as the large and small intestines, kidneys, bladder, and lungs.

Alpha Receptor Dominant	Beta Receptor Dominant
Brain and nerves	Brain and nerves
Blood vessels	Blood vessels
Breast	Bone
Uterus	Lungs
	Intestines
	Ovaries
	Urogenital tract
	Prostate (men)
	Testes (men)

The discovery of the beta receptor is of immediate clinical importance to women, because cancer specialists biopsy breast tumors for the presence of estrogen receptors to see if the cells are likely to be inhibited from growth by estrogenlike drugs. If estrogen receptors are absent, there is no point in using estrogenlike drugs. But present-day biopsies are designed to find only the alpha receptor. If solely betas are present, a false result may be given that no receptors exist, and a possibly life-saving therapy will not be tried.

It is plainly a misconception to think of estrogen only as a female hormone or even as a sex hormone. Any hormone having receptors in as many organs as estrogen has must be thought of as one of the body's main chemical messengers. When the *New York Times* asked Dr. Katzenellenbogen if there was any part of the body that estrogen did not affect, she replied, "I used to think so. Now I have my doubts. Well, maybe the spleen."

It is not known whether alpha and beta receptors ferry their hormone messages to the same or different genes in the cell DNA. But the receptors show some differences in their receptivity to various kinds of estrogen and estrogenlike substances. For example, although alpha and beta resemble each other in strongly accepting the estradiol type of estrogen, the beta is ten times more efficient at binding with genistein, a plant estrogen. Genistein, found in soybeans, kudzu root and, to a lesser degree, the cabbage family, protects tissue against cancer. It may do so by occupying receptors and thus preventing more cell-growth-stimulating types of estrogen from finding receptors.

Both alpha and beta receptors have been found in the linings of blood vessels. While estrogen has long been credited as beneficial for cardiovascular health, its effects were thought to be indirect, most notably through its influence on liver manufacture of cholesterol. The presence of two kinds of receptors in the linings of blood vessels suggests a much more direct role for estrogen in cardiovascular health.

Margaret

At forty-three, Margaret had three teenaged daughters, the oldest of whom was nineteen. She had returned to her career as a chartered accountant when the youngest started school. Her husband and she were happily married, shared a relatively high joint income, and had a lovely home in a good neighborhood. About a month after her forty-third birthday, acute depression hit Margaret out of nowhere.

She had known what it was like to have the blues from time to time and had mourned the deaths of both her beloved parents. This depression was nothing like grieving or having the blues. It hit her so strongly, its impact felt almost physical as well as emotional. It felt like a giant hand pressing her down, and it came and went unpredictably. When it went, it was never far away. Over the next three months her depression became so debilitating that she had to take a leave of absence from her accounting firm.

A psychologist thought at first that there must be some significance to her turning forty-three. When nothing came of that, he decided she must be jealous of her daughters. She next saw a psychiatrist, who tried out different kinds of antidepressants, none of which made her feel much better. Margaret quit when the psychiatrist referred to her depression as a "mental disorder."

One evening, Margaret was lying on her bed with the lights out and door closed, feeling bad and increasingly desperate, when her eldest daughter knocked on the door and came in. Without any explanation, she handed her mother a bottle of black cohosh pills and a glass of water. Margaret swallowed two pills, and her daughter left the room.

Next day, Margaret not only felt better, she also sensed that her body had changed for the better somehow. She asked her daughter about the pills, but the nineteen-year-old was evasive. She said that a friend had given it to her. Finally, Margaret discovered that black cohosh was an herb for perimenopause.

"I think you feel bad because of your hormones," her daughter said. "My friends think so, too," she added defensively.

Margaret couldn't help smiling at the thought of the serious conversations that her daughter and friends must have been having about her. It had been a long time since she had smiled. And Margaret knew immediately that they were right. Why hadn't this occurred to her?

"Where did you get the pills?" she asked her daughter.

"From my girlfriend's mother who went to see this person who's a nutritionist who helped someone else's mother who was even worse off than you are."

Margaret looked at her daughter in amazed gratitude.

When she came to see me the following day, Margaret related her story. We discussed how black cohosh had made such an immediate difference to her emotional state. I explained to her how perimenopausal hormonal changes can affect mood and depression, and how her dramatic results indicated that she was on the right track.

After saliva tests, a few visits, and a few months on black cohosh and progesterone cream, I came to the conclusion that Margaret's symptoms of depression, although much better, were still prevalent. At my suggestion, she consulted a physician, who agreed to put her on a low-dose of *natural* hormone replacement therapy (explained below). Margaret also began using vitamin E as a complementary therapy, which in time enabled her to further reduce her dosage of natural hormones. Keeping the dosage down kept the body more receptive to possible later higher doses if the depression got worse. This can be an important option to reserve. Luckily the combination of natural hormones and vitamin E did the trick.

It is important not to underestimate the seriousness of some perimenopause symptoms. Some symptoms, if ignored, can give rise to whole series of new symptoms. And the longer we put up with untreated symptoms, the harder they are to get rid of when we finally decide to do something about them. Depression is a particularly debilitating condition, because it causes us to be *vulnerable* to many physical ailments.

Soy Phytoestrogen and Phytonutrients

Women in Asia generally do not have the perimenopause problems of Western women. This has led, naturally, to questions about dietary differences. Asian women consume large amounts of soy products compared with Western women, who consume almost none. Soy contains phytoestrogens and other phytonutrients and has been known for centuries to be good for human health.

At the American Heart Association's annual scientific meeting in 1996, in New Orleans, Dr. Gregory Burke of Bowman Gray School of Medicine in Winston-Salem reported on a study that involved forty-three women aged forty-five to fifty-five who suffered hot flashes or night sweats on a daily basis. For six weeks they mixed 20 grams of powdered soy with their food each day, and for another six weeks they mixed 20 grams of powdered carbohydrates instead. The women didn't know which they were taking. The women taking the soy reported significantly less intense symptoms, although there was no drop in their frequency. However, a British study at the University of Manchester did find a drop in frequency with soy. Canadian studies of Japanese women reported soy's success in combating hot flashes.

It is thought that the phytoestrogens in soy—its isoflavones—are about a thousand times less powerful than human estrogen. They are accepted by human cell estrogen receptors, and thus they satisfy the body's estrogen needs and thereby alleviate symptoms. The good news about phytoestrogens is that they have not been connected to breast or uterine cancer.

Soy foods may be either fermented or nonfermented. Soybeans, soy nuts, soy sprouts, soy flour, soy milk, and tofu are all nonfermented. The fermented soy foods include miso, tempeh, soy sauce, and natto.

Some experts believe that the fermented state is the only healthful form of soy. Health researchers Mary Enig, Ph.D. and Sally Fallon stated, in the September 1995 issue of *Health Freedom News,* that unfermented soy products, with their cargo of phytates (an organic acid that blocks absorption of calcium, magnesium, iron, and especially zinc), enzyme inhibitors, rancid fatty acids, and altered proteins, are unfit for human consumption. Fermented or not, soy products have the drawback of being highly allergenic due to the protein and fiber they contain, and they are also high in copper. Additionally, according to the Huntington Breast Cancer Action Coalition of Melville, New York, the soybeans that you eat may have been genetically engineered to withstand high doses of Monsanto's herbicide Roundup. But you can purchase isoflavone supplements that contain the phytoestrogens of soy without the rest of soy's downside. Many companies offer as supplements the concentrates of the primary soy isoflavones genistein, daidzein, and equol, including the following:

EasySoy, from Carlson

Iso-Gen, from Bio Nutritional Formulas

Phyto-EST, from BioTherapies

Essential Woman, from Barlean's

If you don't care for a soy isoflavone supplement, you can try the herb black cohosh. The roots and rhizome of the forest plant black cohosh (*Cimifuga racemosa*) provide a phytoestrogen and a biologically active ingredient that dilates blood vessels. This phytoestrogen relieves many symptoms, especially cramps, irritability, and depression. Enzymatic Therapy produces a standardized extract of black cohosh known as Remifemin. In the July 1997 issue of *Whole Foods,* Dr. Judy Christianson stated that in a recent double-blind study, Remifemin was more effective than Premarin in dealing with anxiety, depression, and vaginal dryness. Madis Botanicals markets a standardized black cohosh extract for women called CimiPure.

Other phytoestrogen-containing herbs that have been used for centuries to balance the hormonal system include dong quai,

---

Ann Louise's
All-Star Peri Zapper #9

Soy Phytoestrogens

If you are in later perimenopause and would like the health benefits of soy phytoestrogens without the possible allergic response to soy foods, try a soy isoflavone supplement.

raspberry leaves, chasteberry (Vitex), wild yam, rehmannia, and licorice root. They can be found in your local health food store as tablets, tinctures, creams, or sublingual drops made by firms such as Phillips Nutritionals (with its highly effective Yamcon line), Born Again, Transitions for Health, Country Life, SunSource, Source Naturals, Rainbow Light, Nature's Herbs, and Zand Herbal Formulas.

Soy Phytoestrogens and Phytonutrients

Phytoestrogens (Isoflavones)
Genistein, daidzein, and glycitein are believed to block estrogen receptors and thereby relieve perimenopause symptoms. They all inhibit enzymes involved in the growth of cancer cells. Genistein can block cancer at several stages and can even return precancerous cells to a healthy state. They are found in soybeans, kudzu root and, to a lesser degree, the cabbage family.

Phytosterols
These help stop cells from proliferating and are particularly effective against skin and colon cancer. They are found in flaxseed oil, fenugreek, wheat germ, and rice bran oil.

Phytic Acid (Phytates)
These phosphorus-containing compounds are powerful antioxidants. They are found in soybeans, wheat, rice, lima beans, sesame seeds, and peanuts.

Saponins
These compounds are antioxidants, prevent cell mutations, and help lower blood cholesterol levels. They are found in beans and other legumes.

Protease Inhibitors
These block the action of protease enzymes in causing cancer and other diseases. They are found in nuts, seeds, and soy.

Foods Containing Phytoestrogens

Alfalfa

Apples

Asparagus

Barley

Beans

Carrots

Cereals

Cherries

Corn

Fennel

Garlic

Green pepper

Hops

Legumes

Licorice

Linseed

Milk

Oats

Olive oil

Onions

Pears

Peas

Pomegranate

Rice bran

Rye

Sea vegetables, dried

Sunflower seeds

Sweet potato

Soy products

Squash

Wheat germ

Chapter 11

Safe Estrogen Replacement Therapy

More Help for Hot Flashes, Insomnia, and Depression

Estrogen replacement therapy and hormone replacement therapy become major concerns during the later years of perimenopause, when hot flashes, moodiness, and vaginal dryness really start to assert themselves and cause discomfort. Both estrogen replacement therapy and hormone replacement therapy are currently topics of heated debate. Any opponent of my views could immediately point out that, as a nutritionist, I am outside my field of expertise when it comes to estrogen or hormone replacement therapy. If I had fewer women clients, I would readily agree. As a nutritionist, I have spent many years helping women overcome side effects from all kinds of medications. As they described the physical and emotional discomfort caused by medications, I listened carefully. Over the years, I have heard a lot about the problem of replacing hormones from the women who have tried it.

I believe that most women are simply not aware of natural options to synthetic hormones. Nor, unfortunately, are some physicians, as I rediscovered for myself only the other day. While I was reviewing material on hot flashes for the writing of this book, guess what? I suddenly had a hot flash myself, followed by another a few hours later. I went to see a doctor. She had never heard of anyone having psychosomatic hot flashes from reading about them, although she did not rule out that possibility. It was far more likely, in her opinion, that my hot flashes were the real thing. I might have speeded their arrival by writing about them, but now they had come to visit and I was getting a chance to meet them firsthand. From what I've experienced so far, I can tell you that if you've never had hot flashes, you're not missing anything, believe me.

I was a new patient, and the doctor didn't ask why I had been reading about hot flashes and had no idea that I knew anything about estrogen replacement from natural sources. She told me it was time for estrogen. By this, of course, she meant horse estrogen. I raised the question of the risk of breast cancer from this kind of therapy. She said—I swear—not to worry about it; even if it happened, all I would need would be a little radiation or perhaps a lumpectomy, and I'd be as good as new.

If a client had told me this story, I'd have disregarded it as exaggeration or misunderstanding on her part. I am not exaggerating, and there was no misunderstanding—on my part, at least.

Hormone Replacement Therapy

Premarin, for estrogen replacement, is the most widely prescribed drug in America today. This can be seen, from one perspective, as recognition by the medical profession, finally, that health issues special to women are as important as those that affect only men.

Or it can be interpreted as exploitation of American women by pharmaceutical companies that see them as their best customers and study their concerns and purchasing patterns.

Susan Reverby, a professor of women's studies at Wellesley College, told the *New York Times,* "As a lasting legacy of the women's movement, health care is one of our shining moments." In talking of medical practitioners, she said, "There's much more consciousness about what women's issues are."

But Rachel Fruchter, an associate professor of obstetrics and gynecology at the State University of New York Health Science Center in Brooklyn, told the same reporter that she was appalled at the way pharmaceutical companies pursued women as consumers. She said, "The pretense that that's what the women's health movement wanted is a bad joke."

As with many big issues, when it comes to hormone replacement therapy, there seems to be room here for equally valid but opposing points of view. There's no doubt that women's health issues now occupy a place of prominence denied to them only a few years ago. To expect this change to have taken place for solely altruistic reasons would be naive. In our society, we expect financial reward for achievement, and there's no reason why physicians or pharmaceutical companies should be an exception to this. Yet no one exposed to today's continual barrage of ads for women's health products could reasonably deny that manipulation of women's health worries is a major selling tool. When selling health products to women takes precedence over providing the health care actually needed, it's fair to say that a line has been crossed. How often does this line get crossed, and who crosses it? Knowledgeable people who are both sincere and honest will give you very different answers to those questions.

My view is that both women and their health care providers are frequently stampeded into expensive major therapy in many instances when an inexpensive minor remedy would have sufficed. This is not always the result of a cold-blooded marketing strategy. We all—patients, physicians, pharmaceutical companies—have unreasonable expectations that laboratory drugs will cure our ills.

Hormone replacement therapy may appear to be the easy way out. If it were, believe me, I would be telling you so in large type. But synthetic hormone replacement therapy has side effects, some of which are extremely dangerous. And the longer you stay on any drug therapy, the greater the chance of side effects. Hormone replacement therapy is not a short-term cure. You are on it for life. The longer you have been on it, the more you need to keep looking back over your shoulder to see what may be sneaking up with you.

Risks of Overmedication with Hormone Replacement Therapy

Blood clots	Headaches
Breast cancer	Nausea
Breast tenderness	Sexual desire loss
Depression	Uterine cancer
Fatigue	Vaginal bleeding
Fibroids	Vomiting
Gallstones	Weight gain
Hair loss	Yeast infection

Premarin and Provera

For relief from hot flashes, night sweats, insomnia, or depression, many women reach out in desperate need for hormone replacement therapy. It certainly sounds good. The trouble for many women is that it doesn't feel good. Even when such therapy successfully alleviates perimenopause symptoms, many women claim that they still don't feel right. There is good reason for them to feel this way. Neither the estrogen nor the progesterone that they take on synthetic hormone replacement therapy is identical to women's natural hormones.

The dominant (by far) commercial brand of estrogen, Premarin was first approved for sale in America in 1942. More than 6 million women worldwide take this drug, with annual sales worth more than $850 million to Wyeth-Ayerst Pharmaceuticals. The manufacturer claims that a total of more than 30 billion tablets have been prescribed. More than 22 million prescriptions were written for Premarin in the United States in 1996. Premarin is a conjugated equine estrogen, which is another way of saying that it is made from the urine of pregnant mares.

The major danger of using Premarin *alone* is its ability to cause cancer of the uterine lining (endometrium). As stated in a warning label on the product, women who take Premarin have a 4.5 to 13.9 times greater risk of uterine cancer than women who don't take hormones. These statistics are further supported by the finding that the incidence rates of uterine cancer have increased sharply since 1969 in eight different areas of the United States. This, of course, is the time frame in which Premarin became very widely used. Other brands have much the same risk of uterine cancer.

Taking artificial progesterone (progestin) was found to greatly reduce or cancel out Premarin's ability to cause uterine cancer. Provera is the most popular brand name of the artificial progesterones. So women are now taking a second drug to counteract some of the carcinogenic effects of the first drug. But not all its effects. Provera does not stop Premarin from causing breast cancer. We will look further at this risk in Chapter 16. It's enough to say now that if you know you already have a risk factor for breast cancer, such as a close family member who has had it, you should not take Premarin.

But Provera creates another problem. It contains medroxyprogesterone acetate (MPA), a derivative of progesterone and a substance with a cardiovascular risk. Kent Hermsmeyer and colleagues at the Oregon Regional Primate Center in Beaverton removed the ovaries of eighteen rhesus monkeys to simulate menopause and gave them daily doses of estrogen. Six also received doses of natural progesterone, and another six received doses of MPA.

After a month, the researchers injected all eighteen monkeys with two chemicals that make the body respond as if it is having a heart attack. In the monkeys on estrogen and MPA, this injection caused an unrelenting constriction of the coronary artery, cutting off the flow of blood. Had they not received treatment immediately, the monkeys would have died. The same thing happened to monkeys not on hormone therapy.

Monkeys that received doses of estrogen alone or estrogen with natural progesterone quickly recovered from the injection without treatment. This seems attributable to the cardiovascular benefits of estrogen. If this is so, it appears that MPA cancels out the cardiovascular benefits of estrogen therapy. That is, Provera cancels out the cardiovascular benefits of Premarin.

Peter Collins and colleagues at the National Heart and Lung Institute in London obtained similar results in tests on sixteen women. J. Koudy Williams and co-workers at Wake Forest University's Bowman Gray School of Medicine in Winston-Salem, in experiments on monkeys, found that MPA can "obliterate the beneficial effects of estrogen on the progression of coronary artery atherosclerosis."

Option: Osteoporosis and Hormone Replacement Therapy

What if your doctor is adamant about your having hormone replacement therapy? Or what if, for some reason, you can't obtain natural hormones? You might consider a new option—having hormone replacement therapy not for the rest of your life but only when it can benefit you most.

Women who start hormone replacement therapy in their sixties instead of in their fifties get most of the osteoporosis-fighting and cardiovascular benefits and very much less of the risk of breast cancer.

"Sixty-five is a great age to start hormone replacement therapy for osteoporosis," Bruce Ettinger, a researcher at Kaiser Permanente and the University of California at San Francisco, told *Health* magazine. This is because women who start hormone replacement therapy in their sixties have very nearly the same bone density as women who began hormone replacement therapy at menopause (according to a 1997 University of California at San Diego study). Fatal hip fractures usually occur around the age of eighty, and starting hormone replacement therapy in your sixties halves the risk of ever breaking a hip.

Differences Between Estrogen and Premarin

Why is Premarin much more likely to cause cancer than a woman's own estrogen? The answer may lie in the different kinds and proportions of estrogen of which both are made up. The following table compares the estrogens found in women's bodies with those found in Premarin.

Estrogen Type	Women	Premarin
Estriol	60–80%	
Estrone	10–20%	75–80%
Estradiol	10–20%	5–20%
Equilin and other horse estrogens		5–15%

Human estrogen is composed mostly of estriol, which is regarded as a "weak" estrogen that does not cause cells to proliferate as readily as many of kinds of estrogen. (Cancer, of course, consists of the uncontrolled proliferation of cells.) Estrone, the main estrogen type in Premarin, is a much stronger stimulant of cell growth than estriol.

The estrogen patch Estraderm and the estrogen cream Estrace are made up completely of the even stronger estradiol, which makes up only 10 to 20 percent of a woman's natural estrogen. Additionally, the lack of a mixture of estrogen types makes the patch and cream even further removed from nature.

Does Premarin Really Cause Breast Cancer?

Most gynecologists with whom I have discussed the question of whether or not Premarin causes breast cancer do not take an official stand. They point to contradictory findings from research on the question. But when I ask what they advise in their own clinical practice, they respond in unfailing unison: do not take Premarin if you believe you have a risk factor for breast cancer. (Yes, it bears repeating!)

The contradictory research findings to which the gynecologists refer are those published by two leading American medical journals in 1995. Graham A. Colditz and colleagues at the Harvard Medical School, in the Nurses Health Study, followed the health of 122,000 nurses from 1976. The study results, published in the prestigious *New England Journal of Medicine,* claimed that women on hormone replacement therapy had 30 to 40 percent more breast cancer than women who never took hormones. Women aged sixty to sixty-four on hormone replacement therapy for at least five years increased their risk of getting breast cancer by 71 percent and increased their risk of dying from it by 45 percent.

The second study was published in the equally prestigious *Journal of the American Medical Association.* In it, Janet L. Stanford and colleagues reported on a much smaller group of women composed of 537 breast cancer patients and 492 healthy controls. The researchers found no link between hormone replacement therapy and breast cancer.

While respecting the integrity of both groups of researchers, medical consumer advocates like Joe and Teresa Graedon began asking difficult questions about why so little is known about a drug that has been approved by the government for more than fifty years.

Breast surgeon and best-selling author Susan Love says that pharmaceutical companies defend their artificial hormone products by pointing out that one in three women dies of heart disease, while the lesser number of one in eight dies of breast cancer. Dr. Love agrees that these numbers are true for *all* women. But for women under seventy-five, three times as many die from breast cancer as from heart disease. And if smokers are taken out of consideration, six times as many women under seventy-five die from breast cancer as from heart disease.

Dr. Love refers to several studies that show that women on hormone replacement therapy are more likely to develop blood clots and gallbladder disease than are women who don't take hormones. According to her, women on estrogen therapy alone have fourteen times more cancer than women who don't take artificial hormones, and women on combined estrogen-progestin (Premarin-Provera) therapy have four times more uterine cancer.

Pharmaceutical companies, Dr. Love points out, realize that it is smarter marketing to emphasize disease prevention than hormone treatment. Thus they claim that their drugs combat osteoporosis and heart disease. She says that the term *osteoporosis* used to refer only to actual fractures caused by thinning bones in older women. Now the term is defined as low bone density. This is equivalent, Dr. Love claims, to defining a high cholesterol level as cardiovascular disease. Research findings at this time are too inconclusive for anyone to make valid claims that hormone replacement therapy helps prevent either osteoporosis or heart disease in women.

So?

If we waited to make decisions about our health until researchers made breakthroughs or resolved their differences, we might have to wait a long time. To me, at least, all is not confusion. Here are some of the things that make the greatest impressions on me.

- Horse estrogens and artificial hormones (most notably Premarin and Provera) are drugs for long-term therapy.

- Drugs taken over a long time usually have side effects.

- Some of Premarin's and Provera's side effects are life-threatening.

- Why take powerful drugs if milder plant estrogens, nutrients, and moderate exercise can deliver the same results in a more natural way?

- The milder the therapy, the greater the probability that you will have sensations of physical well-being.

Cate

At age forty-seven, Cate could live with waking up and feeling like a boiled lobster, throwing the blankets off, and waking up again a short while later, this time feeling like a frozen shrimp. It was when she started to put on weight for no discernible reason that she panicked. She had always led an active life and watched calories. In spite of carefully counting them now and walking up every staircase in sight, there was no good news for Cate on her bathroom scales. Her first name even rhymed with *weight!*

She guessed that her problems had something to do with her time of life and came to see me because she was "not ready to give up yet." I told this tall, large-boned, very attractive woman, who was still athletic in spite of being about twenty pounds overweight, that she need never give up at any time in her life—and least of all now. She and her husband had split up two years previously and she was now living alone, which she didn't like. I suspected that the stress of the breakup and the ongoing stress of her loneliness were associated with her hormonal problems.

Cate surprised me by refusing to have a saliva test to measure her hormone levels. I went along with this, in the hope that she would change her mind later when she began to feel that she was getting her weight problem under control. I didn't have to wait. She had several hot flashes in a couple of days. Now she couldn't wait to have a saliva test. The results surprised me. Her levels of progesterone and estrogen were both down. She was either much closer to menopause than I had imagined, although she was still having irregular light periods, or some other condition was causing the low hormone levels. I suggested that she try natural progesterone cream and take estrogen in natural form, which her physician prescribed. She gradually built up her hormonal levels and achieved a balance. Her symptoms totally vanished, almost overnight. But she has not been able to reduce either the progesterone or estrogen dose without adverse effects. I would say that she is in menopause, except that she still has irregular periods. I expect that she will have a gentle, symptomless transition on her present dosage.

Having Your Hormone Levels Measured

The result of a hormone levels test lets you know immediately if something is seriously out of line. When you know what your hormone levels are, you can then seek treatment, if you need it, on an individualized basis. The test result gives you a baseline with which later test results can be compared, so that you can monitor your hormone levels over time. When you have a hormone imbalance or low level and start treating it naturally, you should feel your symptoms ease and gradually fade away.

Most doctors test only the levels of follicle-stimulating hormone (FSH) and luteinizing hormone (LH). FSH and LH levels are elevated during menopause but rise and fall steeply during perimenopause. Thus, if you happen to be tested on a high-level day, the lab test result will suggest that you are menopausal. To get an accurate and usable hormone profile, you also need to be tested for levels of estrogen, progesterone, and testosterone. But keep in mind that the levels of these three hormones fluctuate, too, so that a test on one day may yield very different results from another a week later. Because your estrogen level is at its lowest on the day before and during menstruation, don't get tested at this time.

Your hormone levels vary with the time of day as well as with the day of your menstrual cycle. To make a future test compare reliably with a test taken today, the future test should be taken at the same time of day and on the same day of your menstrual cycle as your first test—or as close as you can get to it. Another approach is to take tests on different days of the menstrual cycle, spaced apart so that a more accurate overall hormone profile can be constructed.

Blood and urine tests were the only kinds available until recently. To have blood drawn or to deliver a urine sample usually involves a visit to a doctor's office. A less expensive, more convenient method has recently become available: the saliva test. You can take a saliva test on your own, in the privacy of your home.

The results from saliva tests tend to be more accurate than those from blood tests, particularly for progesterone. Blood tests tend to give less-than-accurate estimates because the progesterone that binds with red blood cells gets discarded along with them before the measurement is made. This is not of great consequence when a powerful drug like Provera is being taken, but gentler, low-dose natural progesterone creams, such as Pro-Gest or Fem-Gest, may be made to look ineffective. Saliva tests, on the other hand, register the increased hormone level when natural progesterone cream is used.

About 95 percent of the hormones are bound to proteins, forming particles too large to pass into saliva. Only 3 to 5 percent of a hormone is in a free, biologically active form—and this is what is measured in the saliva test. But you need to watch out that bleeding from gums or from a mouth or lip cut does not contaminate the saliva sample. Another way for a saliva sample to become contaminated is through remnants of hormonal creams on your hands, face, or neck. If you use these creams, wash thoroughly before taking a saliva sample.

While ten years of research back the validity of saliva tests, they are still new to clinical practice. If your doctor recommends them, he or she will supply you with sample collection materials, instructions, and prepaid mailers to send samples to a laboratory. If you have no health concerns that require a doctor's visit but would like to know your hormone levels, you can order saliva tests for up to four hormones at a time, without a physician's reference, from Aeron LifeCycles (see Resources section under the heading of Salivary Hormone Testing).

Aeron charges about fifty dollars per hormone per test. Test results take about five to seven business days. For interpretation of the results, you may need to talk to a health care provider. Aeron points out that its direct-to-consumer hormone levels tests are not for diagnostic purposes and are meant to be used only to monitor changes in hormone levels. When tests are not ordered by a health care provider and are not for diagnostic purposes, they are not covered by most medical insurance policies.

Taking a Saliva Sample

Taking a sample of your saliva is a simple, noninvasive test that you can perform conveniently and privately at home. Hormones in saliva are stable at room temperature for several weeks and so can be stored before being sent by regular mail to the lab.

Taking a sample simply consists of chewing a sugarless gum to generate saliva, spitting into a tube, and capping the tube. You should fill out the date, day of your menstrual cycle, and time of day immediately, since accuracy in recording these is important.

To establish a baseline for any specific sex hormone, the best time to collect a saliva sample is in the early morning before you eat or drink anything, and before you brush or floss your teeth or use mouthwash.

To assess peak levels of estrogen and progesterone, a sample should be taken during days twenty to twenty-three after the beginning of your last period.

If you are currently on contraceptive pills or hormone replacement therapy, collect a sample just before the usual time of taking the drugs.

Estriol

Dr. Alan R. Gaby called attention to the fact that women can take estriol without an increased risk of cancer. Of the three major

---

Ann Louise's All-Star Peri Zapper #10

Natural Estrogen Replacement

An oral dose of 2 to 4 milligrams of estriol quells symptoms (particularly hot flashes and vaginal dryness) just as well as horse estrogen and doesn't increase your risk of cancer. A 2.5 to 5 milligram oral dose of tri-estrogen has the added advantage of protecting you from osteoporosis.

forms of human estrogen—estrone, estradiol, and estriol—only estriol does not encourage cell proliferation. Considered the weakest estrogen and the only one that has anticancer properties, estriol is particularly effective in combating vaginal dryness. According to consulting pharmacist Pete Heuseman of the College Pharmacy in Colorado Springs, the recommended dosage for estriol vaginal cream is 0.5 milligram estriol per gram of cream. One gram of cream is to be inserted daily at bedtime for one to two weeks, and then two to three times a week after that, as needed for symptomatic relief.

The good news is that many manufacturers are now providing products containing estriol instead of estrone or estradiol. By bypassing the liver, the use of estriol creams and oral micronized estriol ensure that estriol will not be converted into estrone, with its increased cancer risk.

Dr. Alvin H. Follingstad pointed out in an article in the *Journal of the American Medical Association* that estriol can be taken orally without losing its identity. A dose of 2 to 4 milligrams of estriol is equivalent to 0.625 to 1.25 of conjugated (horse) estrogen. It is just as effective in alleviating symptoms, has almost no side effects, and does not cause cancer.

See the Health Pharmacies section at the end of this book for compounding pharmacies that specialize in customizing natural hormones.

Tri-Estrogen

Dr. Gaby noted that estriol's main drawback was that it was not as effective as other forms of estrogen in preventing osteoporosis. Dr. Jonathan V. Wright approached the problem of estrogen replacement from the point of view that a mixture of the three kinds of estrogen normally found in the body of a woman of childbearing age presumably maximizes the benefits and minimizes the risks. He made many tests of hormone blood levels and excretion rates in urine before deciding on a 80/10/10 ratio for estriol/estrone/ estradiol. A dose of 2.5 to 5 milligrams of tri-estrogen remedies perimenopause symptoms.

It may be best to mimic the menstrual cycle by taking tri-estrogen as the estrogen level would normally rise and peak, and follow it with natural progesterone. Those of you who would like to find a medical doctor who will prescribe natural hormones, please look under Resources at the back of the book.

Chapter 12

Natural Quick Fixes for Perimenopause Symptoms

It takes many women three to six weeks to restore hormonal balance to the point where they achieve relief from perimenopausal symptoms. On the other hand, some women report that they feel a definite improvement after barely more than a week. Others may take two months before they can definitely say that their symptoms have abated. In the meantime, while you are waiting for your hormones to stabilize, you may need to find some quick relief for your symptoms.

Here are some remedies that I have found effective, either for my clients or for myself. Remember to read labels carefully and follow instructions. These remedies work well for most women and for other women not as well. Some remedies may work initially and then diminish in effectiveness. If one remedy doesn't work or stops working, try another. Once again, these remedies are stopgap measures to be used while you deal with the problem underlying all your perimenopause symptoms—hormonal imbalance.

All-Purpose

As a general remedy for all the miscellaneous trials and troubles of perimenopause, you might try some of the following.

Try an aromatherapy remedy: massage marjoram, jasmine, or rose essential oil over your abdomen.

Try walnut Bach flower essence or the Rescue Remedy combination.

Eat oatmeal dishes, and use nettles in soup or sauce.

The following herbs and plant foods are particularly rich in phytoestrogens.

Apples

Black cohosh

Celery stalks

Chasteberry (Vitex)

Dates

Dong quai (Chinese angelica)

Elder

False unicorn root

Fennel

Fenugreek

Flaxseed

Honduran sarsaparilla

Kudzu root

Lady's-slipper

Licorice root

Liferoot

Passionflower

Pomegranate

Sassafras

Soy

Avoid: Alcohol, sugar, caffeine, too much salt, and processed, fast-acting or high-glycemic carbohydrates.

Anxiety

Vitamin B$_6$ (pyridoxine) is very effective. Remember to take it with a B-complex pill, because the B vitamins assist one another in metabolism.

Try a magnesium supplement, since a low level of this mineral can contribute to anxiety. See under Insomnia for commercial products.

Remifemin, and CimiPure, the nonprescription products containing black cohosh, are also very effective, as is the herb kava kava.

The homeopathic remedy called Despondency, from Natural Care, provides natural relief.

Breast Tenderness

Evening primrose oil helps three out of four women. Vitamin E almost always helps. Try also the following herbal remedies:

Chasteberry decoction or tincture

Fennel seed and sage tea

Marshmallow

Cramps

Herbs are an effective remedy for cramps. Some will work better for you than others because of biochemical differences between women. If some don't work, try others.

Bilberry extract (20 to 40 milligrams three times a day) or fresh berries

Black haw bark (crampbark)

Chasteberry (Vitex)

Dong quai (Chinese angelica)

Ginger

Kava kava

Raspberry leaf tea

Red clover tea

Squaw vine, often taken with raspberry leaf tea

Strawberry leaf tea

Yarrow

You can also try the cell salt magnesium phosphate (6x), putting four pellets under your tongue every fifteen minutes until the cramping stops.

Remifemin and CimiPure help, too.

Craving for Sweet Foods

Try a magnesium supplement. Such craving is often a symptom of a magnesium-calcium imbalance in your body. See under Insomnia for commercial products.

I have found that taking 500 milligrams of the amino acid L-glutamine twice a day, between meals, takes care of cravings for sweets. Alternatives are:

200 to 600 micrograms of chromium per day

10 to 30 milligrams of manganese per day

3000 milligrams of vitamin C per day

Depression

Eliminate all wheat from your diet and add one to two tablespoons of flaxseed oil daily Eat some protein, fat, and moderate carbohydrates at every meal and every snack. When blood sugar levels are controlled, depression can also go away in some individuals.

The major success of St. John's wort as a cure for depression has become widely recognized. This herb works better than tricyclic antidepressants—and without their side effects. Like Prozac, St. John's wort is a serotonin-selective reuptake inhibitor. However, as with most antidepressants, you may have to take this herb for several weeks before its benefits are fully felt. The recommended dose for the extract is 300 milligrams three times a day of the standardized extract containing 0.3 percent hypericin. Half an ounce of dried herb per day can be taken as a tea or tincture. St. John's wort is available in most health food stores. Photosensitivity is the most commonly reported side effect.

In the event that St. John's wort is not right for you, try chasteberry.

Evening primrose oil and Barlean's Essential Woman (containing flaxseed oil and evening primrose oil) are helpful, too, as is 500 milligrams of tyrosine three times daily. It's also worth checking for a hypothyroid condition.

Fatigue

Cut out sugar, and balance each meal with portion-controlled slow-acting carbohydrates, plus some protein and healthy fats. Barlean's Essential Woman can help restore energy.

Try Adrenal Formula from Uni Key Health Systems (1-800-888-4353) or some other adrenal support, such as Mannatech's Plus supplement. Pantothenic acid (500 to 1000 milligrams per day) or vitamin C (3000 milligrams per day) can be a powerful restorative.

Dandelion, a liver detoxifier, helps in your body's processing of hormones, thereby relieving feelings of fatigue. American and Siberian ginsengs have been used for centuries as tonics for fatigue.

Bee-Alive's royal jelly line is a natural energy extender. Bee-Alive's products are fresh and non-freeze dried, unlike other royal jelly products on the market.

Fuzzy Thinking

Get the sugar out of your diet! The Changing Diet Plan (with its healthful balance of blood-sugar-regulating protein, fats, and carbohydrates) is ideal for combating this complaint, as is natural progesterone. At the same time, it might be worthwhile having your thyroid gland checked out.

As a liver detoxifier, dandelion helps in your body's metabolism of hormones, which does much to clear the mind.

Headaches

Evening primrose oil is an effective remedy for headaches. Headaches closely connected to the menstrual cycle and some migraines are best remedied with progesterone cream.

The herb dandelion is a liver detoxifier, which assists hormones in doing their work and often provides a natural cure for headaches.

Hot Flashes

A Swedish study showed that women can lessen hot flashes by exercising vigorously for half an hour three times a week.

The four best herbal remedies for hot flashes are dong quai (Chinese angelica), licorice root, chasteberry (Vitex), and black cohosh. You might also try a decoction or tincture of chasteberry combined with sage.

An Ayurvedic remedy for hot flashes consists of Aloe littoralis, Asparagus racemosus, Crocus sativus, Sida cordifolia, and Tinospora cordifolia.

Dr. Tori Hudson's hot-flash formula consists of three parts sage, three parts peppermint, one to three parts motherwort, two parts gotu kola, two parts raspberry, one part thyme, and one-half part rosemary.

Dr. Hudson also recommends the following formula:

3 drams chaste tree

3 drams motherwort

3 drams unicorn root

3 drams wild yam

2 drams burdock

2 drams orange elixir

A daily dose of 400 to 800 international units of vitamin E is helpful.

A 1984 study showed that 85 percent of menopausal women found significant relief from hot flashes by taking 300 milligrams a day of gamma-oryzanol from rice bran oil.

Nonprescription Remifemin is a popular and effective remedy.

Pro-Estron, from Neutraceutics Corporation (1–800–852–8581), is a commercial preparation of phytoestrogens that has helped alleviate hot flashes for some of my clients. It is available without prescription at most health food stores and many pharmacies. Another product worth trying is Meno-Fem, from Prevail.

For aromatherapy, try Roman chamomile.

Homeopathic remedies include Lachesis and Sepia.

Insomnia

Too little magnesium in your body can cause you to wake up repeatedly during the night or to suffer from frequent sleeplessness.

Many women have a magnesium-calcium imbalance during their perimenopause. Taking a magnesium supplement may solve your sleep problems.

Magnesium Forte comes in capsule form (available from Uni Key Health Systems at 1–800–888–4353). Each capsule contains 56 milligrams of magnesium derived from a complex source of aspartate, succinate, lysinate, citrate, and ascorbate.

Two MAG–200 tablets, from Optimox (1–800–223–1601), provide 400 milligrams of magnesium in oxide form.

Irritability

Calcium, magnesium, B complex, and evening primrose oil are almost guaranteed to help make your personality a lot less thorny.

Dandelion helps get your hormones working better by detoxifying your liver, which in turn makes you feel less irritable. Or try a decoction or tincture of chasteberry.

Natural progesterone can help, and sometimes so can homeopathic Iodum or a natural source of iodine.

Joint Pain

Glucosamine sulfate and chondroitin can help. The essential fatty acids from flaxseed oil, fish oil, and evening primrose oil are effective. The mineral manganese can also be helpful for joint pain.

Mood Swings

Add protein and the right fats to carbohydrate-rich meals, and include the blood-sugar-regulating minerals chromium, magnesium, zinc, and manganese. Try Barlean's Essential Woman.

Support your adrenal glands with nutrients and supplements.

Evening primrose oil, vitamin C, pantothenic acid, or licorice root can be a mood stabilizer.

The chasteberry decoction or tincture that eases irritability and other symptoms also helps with mood swings.

Periods—Heavy Bleeding

Clean up your diet by eliminating caffeine, alcohol, and spicy foods of all kinds. Stop smoking, also; the carbon monoxide and nicotine can prematurely halt egg production and damage the ovaries.

Natural progesterone often regulates heavy bleeding.

For aromatherapy, massage rose or cypress oil over your abdomen.

The following herbal remedies are helpful:

Lady's mantle tea or tincture

Lady's mantle with an equal part shepherd's purse or yarrow

Cinnamon tea

Homeopathic chamomilla or Actaea racemosa is said to be effective.

Periods—Irregular

Try natural progesterone to balance your cycle.

For aromatherapy, massage your abdomen with lavender or melissa oil.

Homeopathic graphites or Actaea racemosa is often recommended.

Periods—Painful

For aromatherapy, massage your abdomen with marjoram oil. A warm compress placed on your abdomen can bring systemic relief.

Try dong quai (Chinese angelica) tea or tincture, or lady's mantle with marigold flowers.

The cell salt magnesium phosphate (6x) can be helpful. Homeopathic Actaea racemosa is often used.

Avoid: Alcohol and caffeine during the week before your period is due.

Vaginal Dryness

An almost constant vaginal soreness or burning, that makes sex extremely painful is a frequent complaint of women going through perimenopause. Perhaps 80 percent of women suffer vaginal dryness at one time or another. *Consumer Reports* magazine found that more than half of its female readers used commercial lubricants to reduce unpleasant friction during lovemaking. A satisfactory vaginal lubricant—or personal moisturizer, as it is often called—is often harder to find than women expect. Lubricants popular for lovemaking, such as K-Y Jelly, are usually water based, run, become sticky, and dry up quickly.

Oil-based lubricants were once thought to make women vulnerable to vaginal infection or irritation, but this has not proved to be the case in practice. Creme de la Femme vaginal cream has a silky-smooth "natural" feeling and has proved popular (it is available from Uni Key Health Systems at 1-800-888-4353). But keep in mind that oil-based lubricants are not compatible with condom use.

Bodywise Liquid Silk is a great water-based lubricant that never gets sticky. Its advantage is that it contains no glycerin, which is suspected of causing yeast infections in women. Although this is a British product, it is available in American stores and catalogues.

You may need to get a prescription for estriol cream. Many women find it well worth the trouble to do so.

Carlson's Key-E ointment or suppositories work well for many women and are found in most health-oriented stores.

The herbs black cohosh, dong quai, Panax ginseng, chasteberry, and he sho wu are beneficial for this complaint. So, too, are vitamin E and Remifemin.

So, too, is homeopathic Sepia.

Avoid: Dehydrating substances (such as alcohol), antihistamines, and diuretics (including coffee).

Water Retention

Vitamin B_6, taken with B complex, is a tried-and-true remedy for water retention. In terms of diet, watch salt intake and excess carbohydrates. Natural progesterone cream often acts as a natural diuretic.

Another effective remedy consists of shave grass, uva ursi, vitamin B$_6$, and magnesium.

You can also try evening primrose oil or a decoction or tincture of chasteberry. For aromatherapy, try Roman chamomile.

Yeast Infection

Eat lots of onions, garlic, parsley, and live yogurt. Avoid sugar, cheese, white-flour products such as bagels, breads, and pastries, fermented seasonings such as vinegar and soy sauce, pickled foods, and foods containing yeast. These dietary recommendations often relieve allergies as well. Drink lots of filtered water. The homeopathic yeast fighter Aqua Phase is extremely effective.

Make a bath or douche of one part German chamomile vinegar to six parts warm water.

You can use goldenseal externally or as a douche.

For aromatherapy, try a myrrh douche.

For a watery but cloudy discharge, try homeopathic Pulsatilla. For a yellow, burning discharge, try homeopathic Sepia or Carbo veg.

Gy-Na-Tren, from Natren, is a fourteen-day program of oral dairy-free capsules or vaginal inserts.

Yeast-Guard vaginal suppository is also effective.

Avoid: Irritating soap and perfume, pantyhose, and tight pants. Cut back on alcohol, caffeine, and fruit juices.

Part 2

The Changing Diet

The whole point of the Changing Diet is to eat hormone-regulating foods that will also help diminish your perimenopause symptoms. Since this is a balanced diet, it will not cause food cravings. The foods are varied and interesting. You will not have to exercise willpower to stay on the diet. When you begin to feel that your perimenopause symptoms are being alleviated, that in itself should convince you that the Changing Diet may be the only remedy you will really need.

While I am a staunch believer that no single diet works for everybody, the Changing Diet is a great place to begin. It's probably quite different from most perimenopause diets, because you *must* eat fats (as well as moderate amounts of protein) and cut down on certain carbohydrates—even those highly promoted complex carbos such as potatoes, corn, pasta, whole wheat bread, and brown rice. High-carbohydrate meals are not recommended because excess carbohydrates—particularly processed or refined carbohydrates such as white rice or white bread—evoke a rapid insulin response in your bloodstream. As a hormone, insulin promotes the laying down of body fat. But body fat is only one reason to avoid excess carbohydrates. The other reason is that a rapidly fluctuating blood sugar level, besides causing symptoms of its own, makes your perimenopause symptoms worse.

Moderate amounts of protein and good fats in your diet help stabilize your blood sugar level. The Changing Diet emphasizes a balance among carbohydrates, proteins, and fats that helps regulate the balance of blood sugar hormones in your bloodstream. This hormonal balance in turn contributes to the balance of your ovarian hormones.

Just as variations in their metabolisms cause women in similar circumstances to suffer from different symptoms, women on similar diets respond physically to the foods they eat in different ways. This is simply my roundabout way of saying that there's no such thing as one diet that fits all.

Anyone trying to put a diet together today has to take individual metabolic variation into consideration. I've done my best to take into account how the bodies of individual women differ in their physical responses to food. But this is an evolving field of endeavor, and at this stage I would be happy to settle for more marks for effort than for perfection.

In the section called Personalizing Your Changing Diet, which follows the menus, I discuss three aspects of individuality that you can take into account while planning recipes. Do you have a fast or slow metabolism? What is your blood type? What is your ancestry? The answers to these three questions can also explain why certain diets have not worked for you in the past.

But before moving on to the Changing Diet, let's spend a little time on why pure water and untainted food are so vital to your perimenopause health.

Chapter 13

Pure Water and Food

Why Nothing Else Will Do

ood and water contaminants can make your perimeno-pause symptoms worse. I suspect that in some cases con-taminants are as much or even more responsible for symptoms than hormonal imbalance. But it would be pointless to try to assign responsibility for symptoms exclusively to one cause or another, because symptoms so often are the results of several causes together. Impure food or water, by weakening the body, can make it more vulnerable to perimenopause symptoms. Viruses, bacteria, and chemical toxins enter the body through tainted food and water. Today, however, we also need to be more wary of even more complex threats.

The use of steroid hormones and antibiotics to speed the

growth of domestic animals and poultry for the market is one such complex threat. Responsible authorities acknowledge that there is an unknown risk to the public, and this has been increasingly covered by the media. The hormones contained in meat or poultry may include estrogen, further adding to a woman's estrogen dominance or excess.

Many synthetic organic compounds, such as pesticides, fertilizers, and solvents, are another complex threat. They are becoming recognized as potent carcinogens, but other health problems associated with them remain little known. An example of this is the growing danger to all women from xenoestrogens in the environment. These compounds are not really estrogens but resemble them sufficiently in molecular structure for the possibility to exist that estrogen receptors in women's cells might accept them as real estrogen. Xenoestrogens are often found in pesticides, and from there they get into our food and drinking water. Their consequences for human health are as yet unknown.

The phrase "pure water and untainted food" has far wider implications today than it did a few decades ago, when taste and visual inspection were often enough to separate the good from the bad. Some of the most dangerous pollutants today are invisible and without taste. Today we need to know, as much as possible, where our food and water come from and how they have been treated.

How Pure Is Your Water?

Water is considered the universal solvent. It is vital at all stages of life, and, of course, perimenopause is no exception. Dehydration is known to cause fuzzy thinking, also a symptom of perimenopause. Water helps to lubricate dehydrated and parched tissues, as well as aiding the body to eliminate wastes. It keeps your skin glowing and your cells and systems working, and it delivers vitamins, minerals, and other nutrients to all your organs. For your glands to secrete hormones and for your liver to break down and excrete toxins, you need to drink plenty of pure water. How much? Most women should drink about three quarts a day, and it's always a good idea for anyone watching her weight to substitute a glass of water for a snack.

Dr. Christiane Northrup has these suggestions:

○ Have a bottle of pure water in your refrigerator at all times.

○ Drink a glass of water about fifteen minutes before eating to help quell your hunger pangs.

○ Bring your own bottle of pure water when exercising or traveling (especially on planes).

○ Drink pure water rather than soda or coffee, which can leach water from your tissues.

The World Health Organization has claimed that 80 percent of world illnesses would be eliminated if we all drank pure water. But where do you find pure water? It's almost extinct. Turning on a tap to fill a drinking glass involves an act of faith that in most places is not justified by the reality.

While technology has caused most of these problems, it also provides the solution. Water is more easily purified than is food or air through point-of-use conditioning. Unsafe water from city pipes or country wells can be made fit for human consumption inside the home. But we need to remind ourselves constantly that water is not necessarily pure just because it comes from a modern municipal system or a rustic aquifer. In America today, all drinking water needs to be purified in the home.

Chlorination

About seven of every ten people in the United States drink chlorinated water. Many studies over the past twenty years have linked the drinking of chlorinated water to bladder and rectal cancers and also to some cases of stomach, pancreas, kidney, and brain cancer. While granting that chlorination is effective against many but not all bacteria and parasites in water, experts increasingly question the wisdom of trading the risk of bacterial infection for the risk of bladder cancer. Some strongly oppose all chlorination of drinking water. Others suggest a change in its technology, including increased use of granular activated charcoal and bubbling of ozone gas.

Fluoridation

Sodium fluoride has been added to drinking water in America since the mid-1940s to prevent tooth decay. Today, about half the population drinks fluoridated water. In studies ordered by Congress in the late 1970s, fluoridated water caused bone cancer in male rats but not in female rats or mice. Since that time, political and economic interests have clouded the results of other studies. In spite of this, sodium fluoride has emerged as a dangerous toxin and an apparent carcinogen in some circumstances. Enough is known about it to say without doubt that this substance is not suitable as an additive to drinking water.

Bottled Water

According to Larry Laudan, in his recent book *Danger Ahead,* the risk that the next batch of bottled "spring water" you buy will be nothing more than tap water is one in four. Except in a few states, bottled water does not have to exceed the standards of tap water. Standards are higher for imported than for domestic bottled waters. The permissible levels of bacteria in bottled water are a generous half million bacteria per liter. Carbonated bottled water is likely to have a lower bacteria count than still water, because carbonation makes the water more acid, which kills bacteria. If the water comes in plastic bottles, plastic toxins may have leached into the water.

Distilled Water

It might seem that distilled water should be the safest of all to drink. Just the opposite may be true. The process of distillation can vaporize and concentrate chloroform and some other dangerous compounds. Distilling also removes essential trace minerals from water. For water to be pure, it must be double distilled. Few companies do this.

Hard Water

For water to taste and look good and also to wash well and not clog pipes, its hardness should not exceed four grains per gallon. Hard—that is, highly mineralized—water was once believed to be good for our health. While it does contain essential trace minerals, its hardness is usually due chiefly to calcium carbonate, which our bodies need but cannot absorb in a desirable way from water. The calcium carbonate contributes to the blocking of our arteries and to arthritis, rheumatism, gout, and indigestion. It may also lead to bladder cancer or heart disease.

Treating Water at Home

My recommendation for water treatment is to use the Doulton ceramic water filter. This is the most effective water filter system available. The filter is made of ultrafine ceramic with pores so small that they trap bacteria, parasites, and particles down to 0.5 microns in size. Unlike some other filter systems, the Doulton system does not create an environment for bacterial growth inside itself.

The Doulton filtering method consists of three stages. In the first stage, the tiny pores in the ceramic remove bacteria, parasites, rust, and dirt. The second filter stage is composed of high-density matrix carbon, which reduces chlorine, pesticides, and other chemicals. In the third stage, a heavy-metal-removing compound reduces lead and copper.

One advantage of the Doulton filter over water distillation is time; it can take up to six hours to distill a gallon of water. An advantage over reverse osmosis systems is that the Doulton filter doesn't waste water, while reverse osmosis systems use three gallons to produce one gallon of drinkable water. The Doulton filter retains its maximum effectiveness for up to 1200 gallons of water. On average, a family of four would need to change its Doulton filter only once a year. The ceramic cartridge can be removed at any time and given a light scrubbing.

You can get more information about or order a Doulton ceramic water filter from Uni Key at 1–800–888–4353.

In Search of Untainted Food

Three federal agencies, the Food and Drug Administration, the Environmental Protection Agency, and the U.S. Department of Agriculture, set and enforce a huge array of regulations to try to ensure that what we eat and drink does not harm us. Like all vast undertakings, this one has its successes and failures, including among the latter some oversights, overlaps, areas of controversy, conflicts, and bewildering behavior.

Food-Borne Illnesses

In the late summer of 1997, national attention was attracted when an Arkansas company was forced to withdraw huge quantities of frozen beef patties because of possible contamination by Escherichia coli bacteria. Although this was an economic disaster for those involved, it focused the attention of an entire nation on the dangers of food-borne illnesses. It is now estimated that in the United States each year, E. coli and other bacteria cause more than 81 million cases of illness.

Most bacteria, parasites, and viruses in food can be destroyed by adequate cooking (from 140°F to 212°F). Proper cooking habits can virtually eliminate the risk of food-borne illness. However, various meats, dairy products, and vegetables have different temperatures at which they should be cooked to kill germs. A new cooking system called the Tru-Temperature Health System is now available that comes with a high-accuracy thermometer in the lid that enables you to cook at a proper temperature no matter what food you are cooking. This system also allows you to avoid cooking meats at too high a temperature, which can create carcinogenic heterocyclic amines.

The Tru-Temperature Health System includes a base cooking

unit, temperature probe, glass lid, plain lid, and instructions. It can be ordered through Uni Key Health Systems at 1-800-888-4353.

Some Food-Borne Illnesses

Food poisoning
Salmonellosis
Staph or "ptomaine"
  food poisoning
Shigellosis
Botulism
Listeriosis

Paralytic shellfish poisoning
Neurotoxic shellfish
  poisoning
Ciguatera fish poisoning
Scombroid fish poisoning
Vibrio seafood poisoning
Mad cow disease

Veterinary Hormones and Antibiotics

In a preliminary report on May 8, 1997, a panel of the World Trade Organization announced that the European Union's ban on hormone-treated beef is illegal. For the most part, the American media treated this as a business story and hailed it as a triumph for American free trade. Partway down its account, however, the *New York Times* noted that the European ban had not been implemented to protect local farmers from American imports but to calm European consumers' fears over chemicals in their food. The report added, "American farmers routinely use five hormones, including progesterone and testosterone, to make cattle grow faster and produce more milk." The *Times* did not go so far as to question whether this really was a great victory for America.

Xenoestrogens

If you live or work in an urban or suburban environment, as most of us do, your body is subject to constant bombardment from petrochemical molecules. These molecules are in the air you breathe, the food you eat, the liquids you drink. They come from automobile exhaust, detergents, pesticides, herbicides, PCBs, and polycyclic aromatic hydrocarbons. Their molecular structures are somewhat similar to those of estrogen, and they have the potential to occupy estrogen receptors in your cells. Breast cancer, enlarged ovaries, and premature cessation of ovulation are possible consequences.

Xenoestrogens—foreign estrogens originating outside the body—are a relatively new field of study. The ones that women are most likely to come in contact with are PCBs and related compounds in household cleaners, detergents, personal care products, small appliances, plastics, canned food, and contraceptive creams. PCBs are known to throw estrogen and other hormones off balance. Another major everyday source of xenoestrogens is the pesticides used for lawns and gardens, golf courses, parks, supermarkets, restaurants, and schools.

The xenoestrogens interfere with the body's natural estrogen in various ways. They may occupy or alter estrogen receptor sites in tissue cells. They may interfere with the actual manufacture of estrogen by the ovaries or adrenal glands or decrease the rate of estrogen excretion from the body and cause a buildup of the hormone, with consequent symptoms. Some dioxins mimic estrogen in the body, while other dioxins block estrogen's effects. Some xenoestrogens have widespread effects, and others have a much narrower focus. For example, the fungicide pyrimidine carbinol inhibits the production of all sex hormones, not just estrogen. On the other hand, the fruit fungicide vinclozolin affects testosterone rather than estrogen.

So little is known about these substances that the picture is necessarily vague. But even a vague picture of unsuspecting women innocently using deadly substances around the home and garden is a disturbing one. You do not need to be an environmental enthusiast anymore to see the good sense of using natural products.

Treating Foods with a Clorox Bath

Bacteria, parasites, pesticides, and other contaminants can be removed from food with a Clorox bath. For more than twenty years, I have used these baths for just about all the food that I prepare at home, and I urge everyone else to do the same. It was originally developed by my mentor, Dr. Hazel Parcells, who used the Clorox bath for all her foods right up to her final days, at the age of 106. Despite a similarity of names, Clorox does not contain any clorine. Although it is made by combining chlorine and sodium hydroxide, the chlorine converts into a new ingredient known as sodium hypochlorite. This ingredient eventually dissolves into salt and water when Clorox is used.

Add a teaspoon of Clorox to one gallon of water, being careful with the quantity of Clorox used, since it is such a powerful detoxifying substance. To ensure quality, I use only brand-name Clorox. Place the food in the bath, according to type, for the following length of time.

Leafy vegetables	15 minutes
Root, thick-skinned, or fibrous vegetables	30 minutes
Thin-skinned fruits, such as berries, plums, peaches, apricots	15 minutes
Thick-skinned fruits, such as citrus, bananas, apples	30 minutes
Poultry, fish, meat, eggs	20 minutes

You shouldn't place ground meat in a Clorox bath. But frozen meat can be thawed in a Clorox bath, allowing about twenty minutes for up to five pounds of meat.

Remove food from the bath and place in clear water for ten minutes. After this rinse bath, dry the food thoroughly.

Chapter 14

The Changing Diet Plan

My Changing Diet Plan highlights low-glycemic (slow-acting) carbohydrates, phytohormone-rich fruits and vegetables, protective fats, and quality protein that will help balance your body's hormones. The Changing Diet will not only help to regulate your sexual hormone production but will also aid in balancing your hormonal response to food, which is so critical in keeping blood sugar levels stable. A level blood sugar helps to prevent perimenopausal symptoms like hot flashes, depression, and mood swings and encourages effortless weight loss. Just remember that any diet that does not take into account the effect of foods on hormones is probably doomed to failure.

The beauty of the Changing Diet is the fact that you will no longer have to rely on willpower to eat right. Your balanced blood chemistry will enable you to control those sugar cravings, which lead to a whole host of perimenopausal discomforts. And since the Changing Diet is designed to become part of a long-term lifestyle habit, make your dietary changes little by little. You may begin to notice, for example, that spicy foods, chocolate, caffeine, and alcohol trigger hot flashes. Then, simply avoid the triggering food or drink, and find delicious alternatives like carob for chocolate, herbal teas and grain beverages for coffee, and nonalcoholic drinks like flavored mineral waters.

Or, let's say that you have been staying away from fat due to a lack of understanding that the essential fats are absolutely crucial for hormone production. To get on the essential fat track, you may want to add a daily teaspoon of high-lignan flaxseed oil on your salads or vegetables. And if you are convinced that you are a candidate for phytohormones in the form of soy, try out the soy shake recipe found later in this chapter a couple of times a week. Hopefully you will agree that soy can be an eating joy (the soy-based recipes sure convinced my clients and me).

A basic underlying tenet of the Changing Diet Plan is the importance of eating organic as much as possible. As we learned in the previous chapter, synthetic estrogens and endocrine disrupters can enter your body in pesticides and plastics. So try to choose plant foods that are pesticide- and herbicide-free with the label "certified organic." Also, try to choose animal foods in which the animals have been given organic feed without antibiotics or hormones, and stick to hormone-free, organic dairy products. Some growth hormones fed to animals are actually synthetic forms of estrogen, which can contribute to the undesirable condition of estrogen dominance.

All in all, if you make the proper lifestyle choices, such as individualized natural hormone therapy and exercise, and start to implement the Changing Diet Plan, I promise that you will be empowered not simply to survive but to flourish during the prime of your life—Before the Change.

Carbohydrates

The glycemic index introduced in Chapter 3 teaches us not only that the refined-white-flour carbohydrates (bagels, white rice, sourdough bread) should be avoided, but also that those overly promoted complex carbohydrates (like potatoes, rice cakes, pasta, and cold cereals, for example) should be consumed in moderation because of the insulin response. As you remember, insulin is a fat storage hormone that is instigated by carbohydrate consumption. High insulin levels not only increase hunger but also may lead ultimately to diabetes (the woman's disease) and heart attack, the number one killer of women in this country. Excess insulin can also affect the thyroid, lowering the metabolic rate, which may account for the dramatic increase in hypothyroid conditions among perimenopausal women for which synthroid is a popular prescription. This is why the Changing Diet Plan includes moderate carbohydrate portions balanced with protein and the right kind of fat.

Unprocessed carbohydrates (whole-grain rye, buckwheat, lentils, dried beans) that are moderate to low on the glycemic index provide high-quality fiber that helps to eliminate excess estrogen from the system by lowering blood levels of this hormone. They also provide important minerals like chromium, zinc, and magnesium not found in processed, refined foods. Plus, the fiber component has the ability to tie up carcinogens in our food and acts as a whisk broom in the intestinal tract to eliminate the removal of poisons. The Changing Diet serving portions for carbohydrates can be found on pages 203–205.

Most of the carbohydrates in the plan are commonly found in a well-stocked supermarket or health food store. There is one thickening agent, however, known as kudzu (it resembles arrowroot), which is a potent source of phytoestrogens—especially the isoflavones genistein and daidzein, also found in soy. Kudzu is a great substitute for corn starch and is high in minerals, especially calcium, and easily digested. This ingredient can be found in health food stores.

Like many plant foods, certain cereals and grains as well as legumes and beans contain phytohormones. Some of these are mildly estrogenic and are estrogen-receptor stimulators in your own body. Others are mildly progesterogenic and are progesterone-receptor stimulators. The best strategy is to include a variety of these phytohormone sources in your diet on a daily basis so that your system will have natural dietary support to regulate itself for more or less estrogen or progesterone as needed.

Check out these phytohormone-rich complex carbohydrates, noting, however, that some may be higher on the glycemic index and so should be consumed sparingly:

Cereals and Grains

Barley	Rice
Buckwheat	Rice bran
Corn	Rye
Millet	Wheat (bran, flour, whole)

Legumes (Beans)

Azuki	Pea
Broad	Peanut
Chick-pea	Soybean
Kidney	

Fruits and Vegetables

Fruits and vegetables, and especially vegetables, are major players on the Changing Diet menu. They are powerful sources of antioxidants, vitamins, minerals, phytochemicals (plant-based chemicals) and phytohormones. The vegetables that are highest in phytochemicals, like cabbage, brussels sprouts, cauliflower, and broccoli, contain compounds known as indoles, which help prevent breast cancer by deactivating excess estrogen in the body. In fact, as epidemiologist John Potter of the University of Minnesota states, "At almost every one of the steps along the pathway leading to cancer, there are one or more compounds in vegetables or fruit that will slow up or reverse the process" (*Newsweek*, April 25, 1994). In the same *Newsweek* article in which Potter is quoted, this statement is made: "It is whole foods—especially fruits and vegetables—

that pack the disease-preventing wallop. That's because they harbor a whole mixture of compounds that have never seen the inside of a vitamin bottle for the simple reason that scientists have not, until very recently, even known they existed, let alone made them into pills."

Now you know why fruits and vegetables are such an important part of the Changing Diet Plan. You can't get their "magic" ingredients in a vitamin bottle.

The orange, yellow, and green fruits and vegetables not only are high in the newly discovered phytochemicals, but they also provide the antioxidant beta carotene that is so helpful in boosting immune function. The dark leafy green foods (such as kale, collards, escarole, and broccoli rabe) are high in magnesium, a mineral that is as important as calcium, and perhaps even more so, in building bones and in calming the nervous system to stave off depression, irritability, and palpitations. Nondairy calcium sources include bok choy, broccoli, kale, and sea vegetables such as nori, hijiki, and kombu.

A vegetable serving is about one to two cups raw, or one-half to one cup cooked. Just remember, the higher the vegetable is on the glycemic index, the less you should eat. Conversely, the lower the vegetable on the glycemic index, the more you can eat.

Fruits are limited on the Changing Diet Plan because many women have the tendency to eat them alone—particularly the higher glycemic fruits, like bananas and raisins—without sufficient fat and protein to offset the rising blood sugar/insulin response. All-fruit meals will not only upset your blood sugar level, creating blood sugar peaks and valleys, but also can feed systemic yeast problems and increase triglyceride levels. High triglyceride levels in women are known to increase susceptibility to heart disease even when cholesterol levels are normal.

Because fruit servings cannot be as uniformly standardized as vegetable servings (that is, one to two cups raw or one-half to one cup cooked), I am providing specific portion amounts for the various fruits. The Changing Diet serving portions for fruits can be found on pages 205–206.

Check out these phytohormone-rich fruits and vegetables, noting that some may be higher on the glycemic index than others and should be consumed in smaller amounts, balanced with some fat- and protein-rich foods:

Fruits

Apple	Muskmelon
Apricot	Orange
Banana	Peach
Cherry	Pear
Date	Pineapple
Fig	Plum
Grape	Pomegranate
Grapefruit	Strawberry
Lemon	Watermelon

Vegetables

Artichoke, Jerusalem	Celery
Asparagus	Chive
Bamboo shoot	Corn
Beans (common, seedlings, kidney with pods, immature mung, sprouts)	Cucumber
	Eggplant
Beet	Garlic
Brussels sprouts	Green beans
Cabbage	Lettuce
Carrot	Mustard greens
Cauliflower	Okra
	Onion

Parsley

Pea seedling

Pepper (red, green, yellow, orange)

Potato (all kinds)

Pumpkin

Radish

Seaweed

Shallot

Soybean

Spinach

Taro

Tomato

Turnip

Yam

Fats

On the Changing Diet Plan, I want you to eat fats (the healthful and essential ones, of course). The changing body needs fats in the form of high-lignan flaxseed oil, olive oil, nuts, seeds, and avocado to help balance blood sugar, assist in long-term energy, strengthen cell walls, and, most important, provide the raw material for hormones. The oil that is perhaps the richest of all in phytochemicals is high-lignan flaxseed oil. The lignan fiber found in the fibrous shell hull of the flaxseed has been found to normalize hormone metabolism, thus helping to prevent both colon and breast cancer.

Based upon the emerging research showing the powerful cancer-fighting properties of high-lignan flaxseed oil, the Changing Diet Plan recommends that each and every woman consume at least one tablespoon of this phytochemical-rich source on a daily basis. As mentioned earlier in this book, you can now find a formula called the Essential Woman on the market, which I personally endorse as a rich source of high-lignan flaxseed oil as well as the other essential female oil, evening primrose oil.

High-quality dietary fat is necessary because it slows down the entry of carbohydrates into the system (thus keeping insulin levels lower) and provides greater satisfaction of hunger. Did you know that dietary fat is the *best* blood sugar stabilizer? And, as you know by now, stable blood sugar for the changing body means fewer mood swings, less depression, and greater mental focus and attention.

The problem is that most of us have been eating the wrong kinds of fats for the past two decades—and I don't necessarily mean the saturated fats. The real villains creating our current health problems are not the saturated fats but vegetable oils in the form of fried, oxidized, or hydrogenated fats found in margarine, vegetable shortening, and fast-food french fries. Sadly, most of these undesirable kinds of fats, particularly the hydrogenated or partially hydrogenated oils, are readily found in commercially baked goods, such as chips, tortillas, cereals, and snack foods; many brands of peanut butter; and even mayonnaise. These fats have been connected to heart disease, immune system suppression, and the inability of the body to use the essential fatty acids.

For the sake of dietary fat balance, however, you don't have to avoid saturated fats completely. Simply keep your intake of saturated fats from animal sources and even palm, palm kernel, and coconut oils to a minimum. Surprisingly, saturated fats like coconut oil (which is known to have phytohormone activity) and butter are the best for high-heat cooking, because these kinds of fats, unlike their polyunsaturated sisters, do not oxidize under high cooking temperatures. So when you see coconut, palm, or palm kernel oils listed as coating ingredients on the labels of nutrition bars, Rice Dream, and carob candies, don't be alarmed as long as you are also including the regulating, protective, essential fats in your diet. The Changing Diet serving portions for fats are found on page 206.

Check out these phytohormone-rich seeds, nuts, and oils:

Seeds and Nuts

Almond	Pistachio
Cashew	Sesame seed
Coconut	Sunflower seed
Pecan	Walnut
Pine nut	

Oils

Coconut	Safflower
Corn	Sesame seed
Flaxseed	Soybean
Olive	Sunflower
Peanut	Walnut
Rice bran	Wheat germ

Proteins

Believe it or not, eating lean complete protein in the form of fish, poultry, lean meat, low-fat cottage cheese, eggs, soy, and whey aids in regulating your hormonal response to foods by stimulating the production of the pancreatic hormone glucagon. As you recall, glucagon performs the opposite role to that of insulin; it helps to mobilize stored fat for use as a fuel source. Sufficient protein at every meal also helps to balance sugar, thus keeping insulin levels lower, and contributes to the maintenance and repair of muscles, body organs, connective tissue, and skin. Protein is dramatically connected to the manufacture of hormones, healing of wounds, growth of hair and nails, and production of antibodies.

Animal foods, like organic lean beef and lamb, are ready sources of vitamin B12, iron, and zinc, elements that are generally lacking in many perimenopausal women's diets because of years of "lite" dieting. And don't forget eggs from free-range chickens. Not only do they contain phytohormones, but they also provide the gold standard for protein as well as essential fatty acids that are the precursors for hormones. Eggs are one of only a few sources of sulfur-bearing proteins that are good for the nails, skin, and hair.

Nonfat dairy products, such as plain nonfat yogurt, cottage cheese, farmers' cheese, part-skim mozzarella, and part-skim ricotta, are sources of complete protein as well as calcium. These dairy products are generally tolerated much better than skim or low-fat milk. When purchasing cottage cheese, take a look at the ingredient list on the carton to be sure you're not buying one loaded with preservatives. Brand-name cottage cheeses such as Old Home and Friendship are good choices, as they contain mainly cultured skim milk. Kraft's Breakstone 2% is another good choice; however, it contains some additives such as salt, modified food starch, and natural flavoring. You may want to rinse it carefully under your filtered tap water. Any of these can easily be found at most major supermarkets.

Soy protein in the form of tofu (bean curd usually sold in blocks), tempeh (cultured soy patties), and soy milk are vegetarian protein sources with well-researched phytohormone activity, which has been previously discussed. One brand-name choice for tofu is Mori-Nu, a brand that seems to be better tolerated by even soy-sensitive individuals. Another tofu choice is White Wave, an organic tofu normally sold in bulk, which is also better tolerated by soy-sensitive people.

However, I still must remind you that in some women soy foods are allergy-producing no matter what the brand, with possible allergic reactions including rapid heartbeat, hives, rashes, and respiratory problems. For these sensitive individuals, it may be best to derive the benefits of the soy phytohormones from supplements or pills rather than foods. It is usually the fiber and protein from soy that stimulate the allergic response.

Also note, as I have previously discussed, that soy is relatively high in copper and low in zinc. And due to a variety of zinc-depleting factors, such as high sugar intake, stress, oral contraceptives, and mineral-deficient topsoil, the zinc/copper balance in many people has been turned upside down in favor of copper. It has been my experience via tissue mineral analysis, that many of my vegetarian clients who are overloading on soy as a protein mainstay at each meal have upset the delicate balance between zinc and copper and have become somewhat "copper toxic," which can lead to problems such as panic attacks, hair loss, and hyperactivity or attention deficit hyperactivity disorder.

But for the majority of you who have never even touched soy because it doesn't sound or look very appetizing, I have included some tasty recipes for your sensual pleasure. This is why, in light of the above concerns, there are still several recipes containing soy, although I am aware that it may not be the best food for every body.

The Changing Diet serving portions for proteins can be found on page 207–209.

Sugar and Spice and Everything Nice

The Changing Diet sweetener of choice is an herb from South America known as stevia. I prefer this sweetener above all others because stevia not only tastes sweet but also can help to naturally regulate blood sugar, is noncaloric, and best of all does not promote the growth of yeast that is so prevalent in three out of four women. No other sweetener that I am aware of can make all of these perimenopausal health claims.

While doing research for this book, I discovered one of the finest quality stevia lines on the market, known as Stevita, which is available in many health food stores. Stevia comes in packets for use at home or when eating out and in liquid form ready to use. Stevita-brand stevia is used in many of the Changing Diet recipes.

Seasonings

Salt contributes to the satisfying taste of many of our favorite foods. But excess salt intake has been linked to hypertension, cardiovascular problems, and even strokes. You may want to use the phytohormone-rich spices to reduce sodium intake, and when you absolutely need to use table salt, consider unrefined sea salt and Real salt, which contain trace amounts of naturally occurring iodine and other minerals. Another salt-reducing secret is to substitute a high-potassium baking powder in recipes that call for regular baking powder. I personally use a baking powder made by Featherweight, which is not only hypoallergenic but also free of sodium.

Other brand-name products that provide low-sodium alternatives include tamari (a wheat-free, lower-sodium version of soy sauce that actually contains some phytohormone activity) and Bragg Liquid Aminos.

While it is true that hot and spicy foods like Indian or Mexican can bring on a hot flash in some women, a number of spices contain phytohormones and can help to balance the system. Since the active constituents of the phytohormones often reside in the aromatic oil, you may want to experiment with a mortar and pestle to release these healing substances. After grinding, to protect these seasonings from heat, air, and light damage, store in a tightly sealed container in a relatively cool place away from the stove. I store my ground spices in the freezer.

Do remember that many spices on the supermarket shelf these days are irradiated, so do look for the pure and natural varieties, which specifically state on the label "nonirradiated."

Here is a list of spices with documented phytohormone power:

Spices

Allspice	Mace
Caraway	Marjoram
Cardamom	Nutmeg
Cinnamon	Oregano
Clove	Paprika
Coriander	Pepper
Cumin	Rosemary
Dill	Sage
Fennel	Savory
Garlic	Tarragon
Ginger	Thyme
Licorice	Turmeric

Beverages

If you are prone to those early hot flashes, then it's best that you learn to avoid regular coffee, sodas, and alcohol, because they are known to alter hormonal balance. These beverages are also important to avoid, starting now, because they act as diuretics, removing calcium, magnesium, and the nerve-strengthening B vitamins from the system. Caffeine in coffee and soda also contributes to insulin excess, which in turn will make you hungry, will introduce a craving for a sweet pick-me-up, will interfere with your ability to make stored body fat available for energy, and can inhibit thyroid hormone production, resulting in a lowered metabolic rate. If you still need a lift, then green tea may be your best nutritional bet. Although green tea does contain some caffeine, it is also a source of highly powerful phytohormones as well as antioxidants.

Soft drinks and diet sodas, unfortunately, are not good substitutes for caffeinated drinks because they present their own health hazards. These beverages, because of high phosphorus content, can affect calcium and magnesium in your system, resulting in weakened bones and nerves. The artificial sweeteners that are used in diet sodas, such as aspartame, for example, may actually increase sugar and carbohydrate cravings because of the chemical components of the sweetener. A whole host of other ailments have been connected with aspartame usage. Dr. Russell Blaylock, in his book *Excitotoxins: The Taste That Kills* (Health Press, 1994), says that the use of aspartame destroys neurons and is contributing to the development of brain and nervous system disorders such as Alzheimer's disease. If you would like more information about the dangers of aspartame, send a self-addressed, stamped envelope and a $1.00 donation to: Aspartame Consumer Safety Network, P.O. Box 780634, Dallas, TX 75378.

Instead of caffeinated beverages, rely on pure filtered water or herbal teas or grain beverages like Roma, Bambu, or Cafix. If you need a sweetener, think of stevia, which will also assist in keeping blood sugar stable.

When you reach for an alcoholic drink, keep in mind that alcohol is notorious for causing a rapid elevation in blood sugar. The resulting insulin surge will again increase your appetite and begin that roller-coaster ride of peaks and valleys in blood sugar. If you are going to indulge (and yeast also is not a problem), then choose red wine or beer because they are the alcoholic beverage sources highest in phytohormones. The phytohormones in red wine are derived from the grape skin (not found in white wine) and are known to help reduce the risk of heart disease. The phytohormones in beer are found in the hops. Limit your consumption to an occasional four-ounce glass of wine or twelve ounces of beer, and consider it a serving of carbohydrate because alcohol affects the blood sugar and resulting insulin response in a similar way.

The Changing Diet Sample Menu Plan

The Changing Diet menu plan and recipes were adapted from menus and recipes created by nutritionists Carolyn Brooks, B.S., and Darlene Kvist, M.S., C.N.S., L.N., coauthors of the book *Picture Book for Zone Cooks* (St. Paul, MN: Nutritional Weight & Wellness, 1997). If you would like a copy of their cookbook, you may call 612–699–3438. Their menus and recipes take into account the effect of foods on hormones. You will also find that many of the Changing Diet meal plans contain phytohormone-rich vegetables, fruits, grains, nuts, seeds, oils, legumes, and spices, which are particularly beneficial for perimenopausal women.

Here are a few guidelines to follow before embarking on your Changing Diet.

- Phytohormone-rich foods are italicized for your benefit.

- The recipes in the menu plan marked with an asterisk appear in the recipe section.

- Try to include at least two snacks that contain some protein, carbohydrate, and fat between meals each day. These snacks, by the way, can also become healthful fast-food meals for when you are on the run and can't take time to prepare a full meal. Sample snacks include 1 tablespoon natural peanut butter on celery (Arrowhead Mills provides one of the better moldfree brands); one plain low-fat yogurt; 1/3 cup low-fat Friendship cottage cheese with 1/2 cup pineapple; one high-protein muffin, made with high-protein powders such as Solgar's Whey to Go (lactose-free whey) or Naturade's Fat Free Vegetable Protein (soy-free, all vegetarian), yielding at least 12 to 14 grams of protein per tablespoon. Most of these protein powders can be found in health food stores.

○ Other possible meal replacements include the 40/30/30 nutrition bars such as the Balance Bar, which is currently on the market. Balance comes in flavors like Toasted Crunch, Cranberry, and Banana Coconut. These flavors are not coated with chocolate—a food that sometimes increases hot flashes in sensitive women. A product called Glycemic Balance by Jarrow Formulas is also available in health food stores and can serve as a meal replacement.

○ Drink at least eight glasses of filtered water a day in addition to the herbal tea, green tea, or coffee substitutes that you may consume during or between meals.

○ If you cannot locate a particular menu item or recipe ingredient, refer to the Changing Diet serving portions for carbohydrates, fruits, fats, and proteins for a list of appropriate food group substitutions and their portion sizes.

○ If fresh fruits and vegetables are not available, then frozen is next best.

Sample Week—Day One

BREAKFAST   ¼ cup raspberries
             2 organic eggs cooked in ⅔ tsp. butter
             *Blueberry Oat Muffin (p. 192)

LUNCH   ½ cup papaya
             *Curried Chicken *Cucumber* Salad (p.194)
             2 Wasa crackers

DINNER 4 ounces organic beef (or buffalo) patty
*Tossed *Spinach* Salad (p. 198)
1 ounce shredded cheese
* 1 Tbsp. Healthful Salad Dressing (p. 199)

Sample Week—Day Two

BREAKFAST ½ *grapefruit*
2 whole eggs scrambled in 1 tsp. butter
2 Wasa Lite Rye Crisp Bread

LUNCH * Lentil Salad (p. 195) served with
Fresh Romaine *lettuce* leaves

DINNER * Confetti Turkey Loaf (p. 199)
1 cup steamed broccoli and *cauliflower*
1 cup cooked spaghetti squash tossed with
⅔ tsp. high-lignan *flaxseed oil* and
Cinnamon

Sample Week—Day Three

BREAKFAST ¾ cup *strawberries*
*Tofu Quiche (p. 193)

LUNCH * Spaghetti Pie (p. 195)
Broccoli, red *onion,* and *tomato* salad with lemon juice

DINNER * Lemon Vegetable Fish Supreme (p. 199)
1 baked *sweet potato*
1 cup salad *greens* with
1 Tbsp. *olive oil* spiced with *oregano, garlic,* and *rosemary*

Sample Week—Day Four

BREAKFAST ½ *apple,* diced
2 organic eggs cooked in 1 tsp. butter
1 slice rye toast with caraway seeds

LUNCH * Salmon Loaf (p. 196)
1 cup *asparagus* spears

DINNER * Cajun Beans (p. 200) topped with
1 ounce shredded cheese and
⅛ cup Guacamole Dressing (⅛ cup mashed avocado,
with lemon juice, chopped onions, and cilantro to
taste)

Sample Week—Day Five

BREAKFAST 1 slice whole-grain toast topped with
¾ cup Friendship cottage cheese (placed under
broiler until cottage cheese bubbles) and
¼ cup blueberries and
9 toasted and chopped *almonds*

LUNCH ½ cup fresh *strawberries*
*Fresh Tuna Kabobs (p. 197) over spaghetti squash

DINNER 1 four-ounce Garden Burger
2 cups mixed *greens* tossed with
½ tsp. *olive oil, dill,* and balsamic vinegar
*Tofu *Pumpkin* Pie (p. 200)

Sample Week—Day Six

BREAKFAST   ¼ cantaloupe
Mushroom omelet made with 2 eggs and ½ cup
  chopped *onion*
½ cup diced *celery*
½ cup diced *green pepper*
½ cup sliced mushrooms
¼ cup salsa, sautéed in
1 tsp. *olive oil*

LUNCH   ½ cup fruit cocktail
* Southwestern Chili (p. 197)
2 cups *cabbage* slaw with caraway seeds
1 Wasa cracker

DINNER   * Steamed Fish and Vegetables (p. 201)
Jerusalem artichoke topped with 1 Tbsp. high-
  lignan *flaxseed oil* and *cumin*

Sample Week—Day Seven

BREAKFAST * Tofu Shake (p. 194)

LUNCH   * Fish Croquettes (p. 198)
Red peppers and *onions* sautéed in red wine

DINNER   * Minnesota Turkey and Wild *Rice* Casserole (p. 202)
Green beans almondine

Recipes—Breakfast

Blueberry Oat Muffins (Makes 12 muffins)

1 cup whole-grain wheat flour
1 cup rolled oats

1½ tsp. *cinnamon*
½ tsp. Featherweight baking powder
¼ tsp. baking soda
½ tsp. Real salt
10 oz. Mori-Nu tofu or part-skim ricotta
6 Tbsp. high-protein powder (Solgar's Whey to Go or Naturade's
    Fat Free Vegetable Protein)
¼ cup canola oil
2 organic eggs
4 tsp. Stevita stevia plus ½ cup rice milk
1½ cups fresh or frozen blueberries

Preheat oven to 400°F. In a large mixing bowl, combine flour, rolled oats, cinnamon, baking powder, baking soda, and salt. In a blender, blend tofu, protein powder, canola oil, eggs, stevia, and rice milk until smooth. Stir into dry ingredients. Gently fold in blueberries. Fill oiled muffin tins to top and bake 18–20 minutes.

Tofu Quiche (Serves 4)

Crust: 1 envelope Kashi cereal (seven-grain, high-fiber cereal)
2 cups water
1 organic egg

Preheat oven to 350°. Prepare Kashi as directed on package. Slightly beat egg, and mix into cooked Kashi. Press into oil-sprayed 8″ glass pie pan. Bake 20–30 minutes until mixture is firm and dry to the touch.

Filling: 1⅓ tsp. *olive* or canola oil
1 cup *onion*, chopped
3 oz. ground turkey
1 pound White Wave tofu
6 organic eggs
¾ cup ricotta cheese
3 Tbsp. lemon juice
2 Tbsp. Bragg Liquid Aminos
1 Tbsp. dry mustard
½ tsp. garlic powder
¼ tsp. black *pepper*

Sauté oil, onion, and turkey in small frying pan until browned. In blender, mix together tofu, eggs, cheese, lemon juice, Bragg, mustard, garlic, and pepper. Pour blender mixture into a bowl, and stir in onion and turkey mixture. Pour over cooked Kashi crust. Bake 45–60 minutes until firm and lightly browned. Knife inserted in center should come out clean.

Tofu Shake (Serves 1)

4 oz. (⅓ of a 12-oz. package) Mori-Nu extra-firm tofu
1 cup fresh or frozen fruit, according to taste
½ cup water
½ cup soy or rice milk
2 Tbsp. high-protein powder (Solgar's Whey to Go or Naturade's Fat Free Vegetable Protein)
1 tsp. *flaxseed oil* or
9 toasted *almonds*
4–6 ice cubes (optional)

Combine all ingredients in a blender, and mix until smooth and creamy. Pour into a large glass and serve cold.

Recipes—Lunch

Curried Chicken Cucumber Salad (Serves 4)

16 oz. chicken breast strips
1⅓ tsp. extra-virgin *olive oil*
3 tsp. curry powder
Dash Real salt and *pepper*
1 cup *onion,* diced
4 cups *cucumber,* diced
2 *red bell peppers,* sliced
2 *green bell peppers,* sliced
8–12 cups *romaine lettuce*
4 Tbsp. natural mayonnaise (for instance, Spectrum Lite, with 3–4 grams of fat per tablespoon)

Heat oil in skillet over high heat. Add curry powder. Remove pan from heat and "swirl in" chicken strips and onion. Return pan to burner. Reduce heat; add diced cucumbers and pepper strips. Cook 3 to 5 minutes until chicken is done and vegetables are hot. Pour cooked mixture into bowl and stir in mayonnaise. Adjust seasonings to taste. Divide romaine evenly among four plates. Spoon ¼ hot chicken salad over greens and serve.

Lentil Salad (Serves 4)

4 cups water
1 large *onion,* peeled
6 whole *cloves*
2 cups lentils
2 bay leaves
1 cup *green bell pepper,* diced
1 cup *red bell pepper,* diced
2 cups fresh *tomato,* chopped
1 cup *onion,* chopped
12 oz. cooked turkey
4 Tbsp. *olive oil*
4 Tbsp. lemon juice
Real salt and *pepper* to taste

Bring 4 cups of water to boil in a 2-quart saucepan. Peel onion and insert cloves. Add lentils, bay leaves, and clove-studded onion to boiling water. Reduce heat, cover, and simmer until lentils are firm but tender, 20 to 30 minutes. Drain and rinse with cold water. Discard bay leaves and onion. Allow lentils to cool.

While lentils are cooking, dice peppers, tomatoes, onion, and turkey. Toss together in a large bowl with olive oil, lemon juice, salt, and pepper. Stir in cooled lentils. Refrigerate at least 1 hour (overnight is best). Serve on lettuce leaves.

Spaghetti Pie (Serves 4)

1 pound lean ground veal
2 cups fresh *tomatoes*

4 large organic eggs
⅛ tsp. cayenne pepper, or to taste
1 tsp. Real salt
6 oz. high-protein spaghetti
2 Tbsp. *olive oil*
1 cup *onion*
1 clove *garlic*
2 Tbsp. fresh chopped mixed Italian seasonings

Preheat oven to 375°. Cook spaghetti according to directions on package. In a large mixing bowl, gently stir together eggs, cayenne pepper, salt, and cooked spaghetti. Pour pasta mixture into an oil-sprayed 9″ round cake pan. Press against sides and bottom of pan to form a crust.

Dice onion, garlic, and tomatoes. Add olive oil to skillet and brown onion, garlic, and veal. Remove from heat and stir in fresh chopped tomatoes, Italian seasonings, and salt to taste. Pour skillet mixture into spaghetti crust and bake 30 minutes. Cut into four wedges and serve.

Salmon Loaf (Serves 4)

1½ cups canned salmon
1 cup steel-cut oats
1 tsp. Real salt
1 tsp. *pepper*
1 cup liquid from salmon plus water
2 organic eggs
2 Tbsp. butter
½ cup *green bell pepper,* diced
½ cup *onion,* diced

Preheat oven to 350°. Drain salmon and save liquid. Remove large bones. Slightly beat eggs in a medium bowl and add salmon, oats, salt, pepper, and salmon liquid plus water. Mix well and let stand while sautéing vegetables.

Dice pepper and onion. Sauté in butter until tender. Stir vegetables into salmon mixture. Spoon into an oil-sprayed 8″ loaf pan or 12 muffin tins and bake 10 minutes until golden brown.

Fresh Tuna Kabobs (Serves 4)

1¼ pound fresh yellow fin tuna
¼ cup red wine vinegar
2 Tbsp. green *onion*s
2 Tbsp. lime juice
2 tsp. *olive oil*
1 Tbsp. Dijon mustard
⅛ tsp. Real salt
¼ tsp. *pepper*
1 large spaghetti squash
2 tsp. butter, melted
2 Tbsp. fresh *parsley,* chopped
8 large mushroom caps
1 cup zucchini
½ cup sweet *red bell pepper*
½ cup *onion*

Cut tuna into 1-inch cubes. To make marinade, combine wine vinegar, minced green onions, lime juice, olive oil, Dijon mustard, salt, and pepper. Pour over tuna cubes, cover, and refrigerate 1 hour or overnight.

While fish is marinating, cut squash in half lengthwise, discarding seeds. Place cut side down in a Dutch oven. Add water to 2″ depth. Bring to boil and simmer 20 minutes or until tender. Drain water. Using a fork, remove strands from squash and scoop into a bowl. Discard shell halves. Spoon squash onto serving plate and sprinkle with chopped parsley and melted butter. Keep warm.

Prepare vegetables for kabobs. Remove fish from marinade, reserving marinade for use later. Alternate fish on kabob skewers with the vegetables.

Grill uncovered 6 minutes on each side until fish flakes easily. Baste with remaining marinade during grilling. Serve over cooked spaghetti squash.

Southwestern Chili (Serves 4)

1 pound extra-lean ground beef
4 tsp. *olive oil*

2 cups *onion*, chopped
2 cups *green pepper*, diced
4 cups Roma *tomatoes*, diced
1 tsp. *paprika*
2 tsp. chili powder
Garlic, Real salt, and *pepper* to taste

In a 2-quart sauce pan, brown the ground beef in olive oil. Add onion and green pepper, and sauté until tender, about 3 minutes. Add tomatoes and spices. Cook until heated through.

Fish Croquettes (Serves 4)

12 oz. canned tuna or salmon
2 organic eggs
8 Wasa Original Crisp Bread (Lite Rye), crushed
¼ cup *onion*, finely chopped
2 tsp. dried celery flakes
Garlic powder to taste
¼ tsp. powdered mustard (optional)

Preheat oven to 300°. Mix all ingredients together gently with fork. Shape into 16 croquettes. Bake at 300° up to 5 minutes on a side until evenly browned on all sides.

Recipes—Dinner

Tossed Spinach Salad (Serves 4)

4 cups *spinach* leaves, well cleaned and dried
1 cup *onion*, sliced
1 cup mushrooms, sliced
1 cup fresh *tomatoes*, diced

Toss ingredients together and serve with Healthful Salad Dressing.

Healthful Salad Dressing (Serves 8)

¼ cup fresh lemon juice
¼ cup extra-virgin unrefined *olive oil*
1 clove *garlic,* minced
Dash of oregano, thyme, basil, parsley, dill, cayenne, sea salt, or
  tarragon

Shake oil and lemon juice together in an opaque container with tight-fitting lid. Add a combination of seasonings according to your taste. Refrigerate several hours to allow flavors to blend.

Confetti Turkey Loaf (Serves 4)

1 medium *onion,* diced
½ cup frozen mixed *bell pepper* (red, green, yellow)
2 tsp. *olive oil*
½ cup oats (thick-rolled or steel-cut)
½ cup chicken broth
1¼ pounds extra-lean ground turkey
1 organic egg
1 medium *carrot,* shredded
½ tsp. Real salt
¼ tsp. *pepper*
1 Tbsp. fennel seed or *dill* weed (optional)

Preheat oven to 350°. Sauté onion and peppers in olive oil in medium skillet until soft. Transfer to a mixing bowl and cool slightly. Combine oats with chicken broth in a 2-cup measure; let sit 5 minutes. In large mixing bowl, add ground turkey, egg, carrot, seasonings, and oat mixture. Mix together with hands until well blended. Shape into a loaf and place on baking sheet coated with cooking spray. Bake 1 hour.

Lemon Vegetable Fish Supreme (Serves 4)

1¼ pound white fish (sole, orange roughy, or cod)
½ cup lemon juice

1 Tbsp. grated lemon peel
2 cups zucchini, shredded
⅛ tsp. Real salt
⅛ tsp. *tarragon*
Dash of dried *thyme*, basil, and *pepper*

Preheat oven to 375°. Place fish on oil-sprayed baking dish; cover with foil and bake for 25 minutes. While fish bakes, combine lemon peel, zucchini, and spices in a small bowl. Remove fish from oven; spoon zucchini mixture over fish. Cover and return to oven for another 8 to 10 minutes. (Fish is cooked when it flakes easily with fork.) Garnish with lemon cartwheel twists.

Cajun Beans (Serves 4)

2 tsp. *olive oil*
1 cup *celery,* diced
¼ cup *onion,* chopped
1 clove *garlic,* minced
½ cup *green pepper,* chopped
15-oz. can pinto beans
15-oz. can black beans
16 oz. cooked chicken or turkey breast, cubed
1 bay leaf
1 tsp. Cajun spices
1 cup water

In a 2-quart saucepan, brown celery, onion, garlic, and green pepper in olive oil. Add canned beans, cubed chicken breast, bay leaf, spices, and water to pan. Bring to a boil; reduce heat and simmer 20 minutes until heated through.

Tofu Pumpkin Pie (Serves 8)

Crust:
8 Original Wasa Crisp Bread (Lite Rye), crushed
Dash cinnamon
2 Tbsp. melted butter

1 *apple,* grated
2 tsp. Stevita stevia
1 organic egg, beaten

Preheat oven to 350°. Mix crushed Wasa crackers with cinnamon, butter, grated apple, stevia, and egg. With fingers, press into oil-sprayed 8″ pie pan to form crust. Bake 20 minutes. Cool.

Filling:
15 oz. Mori-Nu Lite tofu
1 Tbsp. Stevita stevia
2 cups canned *pumpkin,* unsweetened
2 Tbsp. high-protein powder (Solgar's Whey to Go or Naturade's
    Fat Free Vegetable Protein)
1 tsp. vanilla
2 organic eggs
½ tsp. Real salt
1 tsp. cinnamon
¼ tsp. cloves
¼ tsp. nutmeg
¼ tsp. ginger

Preheat oven to 350°. Blend tofu in blender or food processor until smooth. Add remaining ingredients and blend well. Taste. Double the amount of cinnamon, cloves, nutmeg, and ginger if desired for added spice. Pour filling into prepared crust and bake 35–40 minutes. Chill. (Filling will firm as it chills.)

Steamed Fish and Vegetables (Serves 4)

4 cups *potatoes* (white or sweet)
2 cups zucchini
2 cups *carrots*
2 cups *green beans*
2 cups *peppers*
2 cups broccoli
2 cups *cauliflower*
2 cups *onions*

4 six-oz. fish fillets
Basil and/or *dill* weed to taste

Scrub and thinly slice potatoes. Bring 1″ of water to boil in large saucepan. Place deep steamer basket in pan. Add potatoes, cover, and steam for 10 minutes. Add vegetables, top with fish fillets, basil, and dill weed. Steam, covered, for another 10 to 15 minutes. Arrange fish and steamed vegetables on four dinner plates to serve.

Minnesota Turkey and Wild Rice Casserole (Serves 4)

1 cup wild rice
2 tsp. canola oil
1 cup *onion*
1 cup *green pepper*
1 cup *celery*
1¼ pounds extra-lean ground turkey breast
9 black olives
8 oz. canned sliced water chestnuts, drained
1 cup wild *rice*
2 Tbsp. Bragg Liquid Aminos
2 cups chicken broth (fat free)
2 Tbsp. arrowroot or kudzu
1 tsp. garlic powder
1 tsp. poultry seasoning
24 toasted *almonds,* chopped

Rinse wild rice and soak for 2 hours in 2 cups of boiling water. Preheat oven to 350°. In a large skillet, sauté onion, green pepper, celery, and ground turkey breast in oil until turkey is brown. Add olives, water chestnuts, prepared wild rice, Bragg, and chicken broth to skillet. Mix together arrowroot or kudzu, garlic powder, and poultry seasoning. Add to skillet and stir until well blended. Bake in an oil-sprayed, covered 3-quart casserole 45 minutes until liquid is absorbed. Spoon onto plates. Garnish each serving with 6 chopped, toasted almonds.

The Changing Diet Serving Portions

Changing Diet Serving Portions for Carbohydrates

Starchy Vegetables

Chestnuts, roasted	4 large or 6 small
Corn (on the cob)	1 (4 in. long)
Corn (cooked)	½ cup
Parsnips	1 small
Peas (fresh)	¼ cup
Potatoes, white (baked or boiled)	1 small
Potatoes, white (mashed)	½ cup
Pumpkin	¾ cup
Rutabaga	1 small
Squash (winter types)	½ cup
Succotash	½ cup

Breads

Bagel, whole wheat	½ small
Bread (rye, pumpernickel, whole wheat)	½ slice
Breadsticks	4 (7 in. long)
Bun (hamburger or hot dog)	One-half
Croutons	½ cup
Pancakes (whole grain)	2 (3″ diameter)
Pita bread	One-half (6″ pocket)
Tortilla, corn	1 (6″)

Cereals and Grains

Amaranth (cooked)	¼ cup
Barley (cooked)	¼ cup
Bran flakes	¼ cup
Bran (unprocessed rice or wheat)	¼ cup
Buckwheat groats (kasha, cooked)	¼ cup
Cornmeal (cooked)	¼ cup

Couscous	¼ cup
Grits (cooked)	¼ cup
Kamut	¼ cup
Millet (cooked)	¼ cup
Oat groats	½ cup
Oats, rolled	½ cup
Oatmeal (steel-cut)	½ cup
Quinoa (cooked)	¼ cup
Rice (brown, cooked)	¼ cup
Rice (wild, cooked)	¼ cup
Rolled rye	½ cup
Rye berries	¼ cup
Shredded-wheat biscuit	1 large
Spelt	¼ cup
Tapioca	2 Tbsp.
Teff	½ cup
Wheat (bulgur, cracked, rolled)	¼ cup
Wheatena (cooked)	½ cup
Wheat germ	1 oz. or 3 Tbsp.

Crackers

Matzoh (whole wheat)	½ (6″ x 4″)
Pretzels (whole grain)	1 large
Rice wafers (brown rice, Westbrae)	4
Ryvita Light Crisp Bread	1–1½ crackers
Ryvita Dark Crisp Bread	1–1½ crackers
Ryvita Original Snack Bread	2 crackers
Ryvita Sesame Snack Bread	2 crackers
Wasa Hearty Crisp Bread	1 cracker
Wasa Light Rye Crisp Bread	2 crackers
Wasa Savory Crisp Bread	2 crackers
Wasa Whole Grain Crisp Bread	2 crackers
Whole-wheat crackers (AK-Mak)	4 crackers
Whole-wheat crackers (Health Valley)	13 crackers

Flours

Arrowroot	2 Tbsp.
Buckwheat	3 Tbsp.

Cornmeal	2 Tbsp.
Cornstarch	2 Tbsp.
Potato flour	2½ Tbsp.
Rice flour	3 Tbsp.
Soya powder	3 Tbsp.
Whole wheat	3 Tbsp.

Legumes

Beans: lima, navy, pinto, kidney, garbanzo, black (dried, cooked)	½ cup
Beans (baked, plain)	½ cup
Lentils (dried, cooked)	¼ cup
Peas (dried, cooked)	½ cup
Peas (split)	¼ cup

Pasta

Noodles: macaroni, spaghetti (cooked)	¼ cup
Noodles: rice (cooked)	¼ cup
Noodles: whole wheat (cooked)	¼ cup
Pasta: whole wheat (cooked)	¼ cup

Changing Diet Serving Portions for Fruit

Apple	One-half
Apple butter (sugar-free)	2 Tbsp.
Apple juice or cider	⅓ cup
Applesauce (unsweetened)	¼ cup
Apricots (fresh)	3
Apricots (dried and unsulfured)	4 halves
Banana	One-third
Berries: boysenberries, blackberries, blueberries, loganberries	½ cup
Cantaloupe	One-quarter melon or 1 cup cubed
Cherries	7
Dates	2
Figs (fresh)	1 large

Figs (dried)	1 small
Fruit cocktail (canned in juice)	½ cup
Fruit preserves and spreads (sugar-free)	2 Tbsp.
Grapefruit	One-half small
Grapefruit juice	½ cup
Grapes	10
Grape juice	¼ cup
Honeydew melon, cubed	½ cup
Kiwi	1 medium
Lemon	1
Lime	1
Mango, sliced	⅓ cup
Nectarine	One-half
Oranges, Mandarin (canned)	⅓ cup
Orange	One-half
Orange juice (any style)	½ cup
Papaya	½ cup
Peach	1 medium
Peaches, canned	½ cup
Pear	One-third
Persimmon	1 medium
Pineapple	½ cup
Pineapple juice	⅓ cup
Plums	1
Prunes	2 medium
Prune juice	¼ cup
Raisins	2 Tbsp.
Raspberries	⅔ cup
Strawberries	¾ cup
Tangerine	1 large
Watermelon	½ cup

Changing Diet Serving Portions for Fats

A variety of nuts and seeds are recommended in this section.

Due to the enzyme inhibitors present in raw seeds, nuts, and legumes, it is suggested that you toast all raw nuts and seeds in the oven for about 20 minutes at 300° to deactivate the inhibitors.

Almonds, raw whole	3
Almonds, slivered	1½ tsp.
Almond butter, unroasted	½ tsp.
Avocado	1 Tbsp.
Brazil nuts, raw whole	2
Butter	⅓ tsp.
Canola oil	⅓ tsp.
Cream, half & half	1 Tbsp.
Cream, light coffee	½ Tbsp.
Cream, sour	½ Tbsp.
Cream cheese	1 tsp.
Flaxseed oil	⅓ tsp.
Grapeseed oil	⅓ tsp.
Guacamole	½ Tbsp.
Hazelnuts, raw whole	3
Macadamia nuts, raw whole	1
Macadamia oil	⅓ tsp.
Mayonnaise (canola based)	1 tsp.
Nayonaise (soy based)	½ Tbsp.
Olive oil	⅓ tsp.
Olive oil and vinegar dressing	1 tsp.
Olives	3
Pecans, raw halves	3
Pine nuts, raw	1 tsp.
Pumpkin seeds, raw	¾ tsp.
Sunflower seeds, raw	¾ tsp.
Tahini, unroasted	1 Tbsp.
Walnuts, raw halves	2

Changing Diet Serving Portions for Proteins

Meat and Poultry (organic preferred)

Beef, ground (10% or less fat)	1.5 oz.
Beef, lean cuts: top round, eye of round, sirloin, sirloin tip	1.5 oz.
Buffalo	1 oz.

Chicken breast, skinless	1 oz.
Duck	1.5 oz.
Egg, whites	2
Egg, whole	1
Lamb, lean	1.5 oz.
Ostrich	1 oz.
Rabbit	1.5 oz.
Turkey breast, skinless	1 oz.
Turkey, dark meat, skinless	1.5 oz.
Veal	1.5 oz.
Venison	1 oz.

Fish and Seafood

Bass	1.5 oz.
Bluefish	1.5 oz.
Calamari	1.5 oz.
Catfish	1.5 oz.
Cod	1.5 oz.
Clams	1.5 oz.
Crab meat	1.5 oz.
Haddock	1.5 oz.
Halibut	1.5 oz.
Lobster	1.5 oz.
Mackerel	1.5 oz.
Orange Roughy	1.5 oz.
Pike, Northern	1.5 oz.
Salmon	1.5 oz.
Sardines	1 oz.
Scallops	1.5 oz.
Shrimp	1.5 oz.
Snapper	1.5 oz.
Sole	1.5 oz.
Swordfish	1.5 oz.
Trout	1.5 oz.
Trout, canned in water	1 oz.
Tuna (steak)	1.5 oz.
Tuna, canned in water	1 oz.

Dairy

Cottage cheese, dry curd (Old Home)	¼ cup
Cottage cheese, low fat (Friendship)	¼ cup
Cheese, reduced fat	1 oz.
Farmers	¼ cup
Mozzarella, skim	1 oz.
Ricotta, skim	2 oz. or ¼ cup
Parmesan	2 Tbsp.

Vegetarian

Solgar's Whey to Go (lactose-free whey)	1 Tbsp.
Naturade's Fat Free Vegetable Protein	1 Tbsp.

Chapter 15

Personalizing Your Changing Diet

W omen vary as much in their metabolism as they do in their variety of perimenopausal symptoms. Although I believe that the Changing Diet is a good place to begin, the truth is that no single diet fits all. To further personalize your needs, I have selected three factors to keep in mind: metabolic rate, blood type, and ancestry.

Metabolic Rate

If you are like the majority of my clients, you are likely to belong to one of two metabolic types: slow or fast burners. Due to their underactive adrenal and thyroid glands, slow burners burn food too slowly, causing them to feel lethargic and tired. They often prefer simple sugars, sweet foods, processed carbohydrates, and soda because of the quick lift these provide. They eat starchy foods to excess. Since their digestion tend to be sluggish, they dislike protein- and fat-rich foods. Slow burners often have poor circulation, dry skin, and a tendency toward diabetes and obesity.

Slow burners need to add enough protein to their diets and reduce excessive carbohydrate intake from pasta, bread, and sweets. Increased amounts of protein will increase metabolic rate considerably, help to burn fat stores, and provide more energy. Slow burners should consume animal protein from lean light sources (such as tuna, cod, poultry, and eggs) at two meals each day and watch their fat intake.

Fast burners on the other hand, possess overactive adrenal glands and dysfunctional thyroid glands, often burning food too quickly, especially carbohydrates. When they lack sufficient fat and protein in their diets, they frequently feel hyper, anxious, or irritable, with emotional peaks and valleys corresponding to energy highs and lows. Fast burners often suffer from hypoglycemia.

Fast burners need to consume healthy fats and purine-rich proteins and vegetables like sardines, organ meats and spinach, for example. At every meal, they should eat some protein, such as venison, beef, lamb, cold-water fish, or full-fat dairy products like cheese and yogurt. These foods slow down their metabolism.

Not everyone is a slow or fast burner. If you tend to put on weight easily, however, it is quite likely that you are one or the other. If you are neither (that is, a mixed oxidizer), your diet should combine features for both fast and slow burners.

Your metabolic type can also be discovered through tissue mineral analysis of a hair sample. Answering the following quizzes (adapted from my book *Your Body Knows Best*) should give you an idea of which general type you belong to. Answer yes or no to each question.

Slow Burner Quiz

1. Do people regard you as restrained and even-tempered?

   ———

2. When you eat red meat, does it feel "heavy" in your system?

   ———

3. Do you prefer to tackle problems one at a time rather than several at once? _____

4. Can you skip breakfast without getting hungry or feeling a loss of energy? _____

5. Do you feel a quick pickup from candy, fruit, and other sweet things? _____

6. Do you prefer a "light" meal (say, salad or pasta) to a "heavy" meal (say, red meat)? _____

7. Do you become thirsty frequently? _____

8. Do foods like butter, cheese, and avocados make you feel sluggish? _____

9. Do you need coffee each morning? _____

10. Do you like spices in food and use condiments like mustard, ketchup, and salsa? _____

Fast Burner Quiz

1. Do people regard you as high-strung or hyperactive? _____

2. Do you feel better after eating red meat than poultry? _____

3. Do you like a "hearty" breakfast (say, bacon and eggs)? _____

4. Under stress, do you reach for salty snacks like nuts or potato chips? _____

5. Do full-fat dairy products, cheese sauces, and avocados give you a feeling of satisfaction? _____

6. Does eating a full meal every three or fours hours make you feel better? _____

7. When you eat sweet foods, do you feel an energy boost and then an energy loss? _____

8. Do you have an excellent appetite? _____

9. After drinking coffee, do you feel nervous or anxious? _____

10. Does butter on toast give you more satisfaction than preserves? _____

If you answered yes to eight or more questions in either quiz, you are a classic slow or fast burner, whichever applies.

Fast burners gain the greatest benefits from the Changing Diet Plan because of the higher amounts of protein and healthful fats already included. Slow burners may need to adjust the fats downward and the carbs upward by, let's say, cutting out a tablespoon of oil and increasing the portions of vegetables, fruits, and brown rice.

If you scored somewhere between slow and fast burners—and are therefore a mixed oxidizer—the Changing Diet will continue to keep you balanced.

Blood Type

An intriguing and important aspect of human evolution concerns the evolution of the four major human blood types and how each represents a somewhat different kind of nutritional need. A leading researcher, the naturopathic physician Dr. Peter J. D'Adamo, has recently published a book on this subject and is considered an expert on the blood type/nutrition connection.

As humans underwent major changes in their efforts to survive in challenging environments, certain adaptive genetic changes are thought to have proved advantageous in new environments. The four different blood types may very well represent such advantageous adaptive genetic change.

Type O is believed to be the oldest blood type, at its peak when humans were at the nomadic hunter-gatherer stage, about 40,000 B.C.E. Type A is thought to have evolved when humans became settled in agricultural communities, from about 25,000 to 15,000 B.C.E. Obviously, a change of diet occurs when nomadic hunter-gatherers become settled farmers. Type A blood seems to have evolved to accomodate a more agrarian diet. If the adaptive genetic change had been disadvantageous, individuals with the new blood type A would not have left descendants.

Blood type B evolved in the Himalayan mountains between 15,000 and 10,000 B.C.E. As these nomadic people later expanded over the Eurasian plains, this blood type became more widespread.

Type AB is believed to be the newest blood group. This blood group seems to have evolved about ten to twelve centuries ago, in an era of trade, new migrations, and conquests.

And so in addition to your metabolic rate, you may want to consider your blood type as another factor to individualize the Changing Diet one step further. Here are some basic recommendations. More in depth information is contained in my book *Your Body Knows Best.*

Type O. A high-protein, low-carbohydrate diet suited type O people for the intense physical activity of hunting. They ate a lot of wild game and whatever wild plants they could. Lean animal protein, free of artificial hormones, antibiotics, and preservatives, is their ideal food in addition to lots of vegetables and some fruit. People with this blood type tend to feel that their bodies do not properly process foods that developed in the later agricultural stage of human evolution. These foods primarily include dairy products (milk, cheese, yogurt), and grain foods from wheat (pasta, bread, bagels). The Changing Diet is good for people with type O blood nutritional requirements, except for dairy and wheat foods. They should avoid dairy foods or use lactose-reduced dairy products or the enzyme product Lactaid. Type O's should eat gluten-free bread made from rice, tapioca, or millet and avoid whole-wheat bread, crackers, and pita. Although spelt and kamut contain some gluten, they may not cause a problem.

Type A. While a typical type O is a meat eater, a typical type A is almost a vegetarian. Type A people need to ensure that their diets are balanced and that they are ingesting enough protein, vitamins, and minerals. About the only thing they have in common with type O people is poor digestion of dairy products. Genetically, type A people tend to lack sufficient hydrochloric acid for effective digestion of proteins. They can accommodate this by eating lighter protein foods and supplementing with a hydrochloric acid and pepsin dietary supplement.

Type B. People with blood type B digest almost all kinds of foods very well, including cultured dairy products. The Changing Diet is very good for people with this blood type as they seem to require some animal protein in the diet. However, type B's should substitute turkey or fish for chicken in the menu. They can eat yogurt and fermented dairy products, too.

Type AB. Some people with this rare blood type resemble type A's in their nutritional requirements, except that they may be able to digest certain dairy products properly. (I would still recommend a hydrochloric acid and pepsin supplement for type AB's.) Others resemble type B's in their nutritional requirements. Generally, this type, because it is the newest blood type, should eat a varied diet of foods from every food group rather than a spartan eating plan.

Ancestry

In the last two centuries, our technological evolution has far outpaced our physical evolution. For example, we now venture into environments in outer space and beneath the sea that we will probably never adapt to, regardless of time. But we Americans are also travelers on a more earthbound scale. Our origins lie among northern European, Mediterranean, African, Asian, or Native American peoples with their own very distinctive diets. It is reasonable to suppose that, to some extent, these various peoples have physically adjusted to their characteristic foods in various ways and are at their healthiest when eating them. If you belong exclusively to some geographic or ethnic group with a characteristic diet, it will probably be beneficial to you to adjust the Changing Diet to fit that diet. A woman of predominantly Italian or Mediterranean ancestry, for example, could use more olive oil, garlic, and legumes as food choices, while a woman of Asian ancestry could substitute sesame oil, sea vegetables, and fish in the menu plans and recipes.

In closing, I hope you will consider some of these factors in developing the perfect version of the Changing Diet for your own unique body chemistry. I also hope that your journey through perimenopause will be totally supported by the knowledge that you can simply, safely, and naturally head off discomforting symptoms by taking charge of your diet and special nutrient needs. May you blossom and flourish during this next stage of life!

Chapter 16

Roundup

The All-Star Peri Zappers at a Glance

For your convenience, here are all ten of my All-Star Peri Zappers. Remember that they are most effective when you use them with the Changing Diet Plan.

Ann Louise's All-Star Peri Zapper #1

Flaxseed Oil

As an all-around peri balancer—especially for skin conditions, depression, and fatigue—nothing beats a daily tablespoonful of flaxseed oil that is high in lignans. Swallow as is or use as a salad dressing or topping for grains and veggies and in no-heat recipes.

Ann Louise's All-Star Peri Zapper #2

Evening Primrose Oil

For breast tenderness, particularly, but also for mood changes, anxiety, irritability, headaches, and water retention, take two capsules (500 milligrams) of evening primrose oil twice daily after food.

Ann Louise's All-Star Peri Zapper #3

M 'n' M (Multivitamins and Magnesium)

Many women's perimenopausal symptoms (such as mood swings, insomnia, anxiety, tissue dryness, and water retention) are alleviated by the following combination of supplements:

- Vitamin B complex, including 50 to 100 milligrams of vitamin B_6
- Vitamin C, 1000 milligrams three times a day
- Vitamin E, 400 to 1200 international units
- Magnesium, 500 to 1000 milligrams before sleeping

When you feel that your hormones are back in better balance, you may be able to cut back to 1000 milligrams a day of vitamin C and to 400 international units of vitamin E.

Ann Louise's All-Star Peri Zapper #4

Think Zinc

Zinc (15 to 50 milligrams a day) helps to lower estrogen and increase progesterone levels, build strong bones, and keep your immune system in tiptop shape to ward off viruses. A must for vegetarians, whose diet is often lacking in this vital mineral.

Ann Louise's All-Star Peri Zapper #5

Natural Progesterone Cream

Progesterone cream balances estrogen dominance symptoms, such as decreased sex drive, depression, abnormal blood sugar levels, fatigue, fuzzy thinking, irritability, thyroid dysfunction, water retention, bone loss, fat gain, and low adrenal function.

Massage a high-quality progesterone cream into the soft, capillary-rich skin of your face, neck, upper chest, breasts, inner arms, palms and backs of hands, and soles. Rotate skin areas daily so that you don't saturate the subdermal receptors. Apply from the twelfth to the twenty-sixth day of your menstrual cycle. Use a total of 1/8 to 1/2 teaspoon daily to start, in one or two applications a day.

Ann Louise's All-Star Peri Zapper #6

Exercise

Be vigorously active for a half hour five days a week. Do housework, garden, walk briskly, cycle, swim, dance, have fun. Do different things each day—and do what you enjoy.

Ann Louise's All-Star Peri Zapper #7

Destressing Stress

Remember that you perceive a stressor as such and that stress is a three-step process:

- Stressor
- Distress
- Consequence

The process can be interrupted at any step.

Ann Louise's All-Star Peri Zapper #8

Adrenal Refresher

At times of a lot of stress, replacing lost minerals and vitamins can help the adrenal glands secrete stress hormones. Try the following:

- B complex vitamins
- Vitamin C, 500 milligrams every three hours
- Adrenal gland extract

- Green and yellow-orange vegetables
- Sea vegetables as a condiment

Ann Louise's All-Star Peri Zapper #9

Soy Phytoestrogens

If you are in later perimenopause and would like the health benefits of soy phytoestrogens without the possible allergic response to soy foods, try a soy isoflavone supplement.

Ann Louise's All-Star Peri Zapper #10

Natural Estrogen Replacement

An oral dose of 2 to 4 milligrams of estriol quells symptoms (particularly hot flashes and vaginal dryness) just as well as horse estrogen and doesn't increase your risk of cancer. A 2.5- to 5-milligram oral dose of tri-estrogen has the added advantage of protecting you from osteoporosis.

Remember to take only the absolute minimum that you need to alleviate your symptoms. And keep in mind that these remedies work in conjunction with the Changing Diet. When they and it are used together, they lend power to each other. I hope they bring you the relief and happiness they have brought to so many other women voyaging through perimenopause!

Selected References

Abrahamson, E. M., and A. W. Pezet. *Body, Mind and Sugar.* New York: Holt, Rinehart, 1951.

Aesoph, Lauri. "Body Wise: Health Alert for Women." *Delicious!,* October 1996, 26–30.

Andrews, Edmund L. "In Victory for U.S., Europe Ban on Treated Beef Is Ruled Illegal." *New York Times,* May 9, 1997.

Angier, Natalie. "New Respect for Estrogen's Influence." *New York Times,* June 24, 1997.

ARHP Clin. Proc. (July 1993).

"Benefits Are Found in Asian Fish Diet." *New York Times,* Aug. 1, 1997.

Beutler, Jade. "High in Lignan Flax Oil." *Health Perspectives* 3, no. 2 (Mar./Apr. 1997): 1–2.

Bland, Jeffrey S. "Back to Basics: Dietary Fiber, Perimenopause and Estrogen." *Let's Live,* Apr. 1995, 91.

Bloom, Marc. "Gain Without Pain: Fitness a Dose at a Time." *New York Times,* June 22, 1997.

Brody, Jane E. "Drug Researchers Working to Design Customized Estrogen." *New York Times,* Mar. 4, 1997.

———. "Trans Fatty Acids Tied to Risk of Breast Cancer." *New York Times,* Oct. 14, 1997.

Caldwell, L. "Is Male Menopause Myth or Reality?" *Men's Fitness,* July 1994, 102–4.

Cassidy, A. *Biological Effects of Plant Estrogens in Premenopausal Women.* American Society for Experimental Biology Abstract, no. A866 (1993).

Christiano, Donna. "Hot Flashes at 39?" *McCall's,* September 1995, 58.

Colditz, Graham A., et al. "The Use of Estrogens and Progestins and the Risk of Breast Cancer in Postmenopausal Women." *New England Journal of Medicine* 332 (1995): 1589–93.

Cranton, Elmer. *Resetting the Clock.* New York: Evans, 1996.

Crayhon, Robert. *Robert Crayhon's Nutrition Made Simple.* New York: Evans, 1994.

Dabbs, J. "Salivary Testosterone Measurements: Collecting, Storing, and Mailing Saliva Samples." *Physiology & Behavior* 49 (1991): 815–17.

D'Adamo, Peter J. *Eat Right for Your Type.* New York: Putnam, 1996.

Daniel, Jill. "The Nutrients You May Be Missing." *Walking Magazine,* Jan./Feb. 1997, 28–30.

Diamond, Seymour. *The Hormone Headache.* New York: Macmillan, 1995.

Duke, James A. *The Green Pharmacy.* Emmaus, PA: Rodale, 1997.

Eaton, S. Boyd, and Melvin Konner. "Paleolithic Nutrition: A Consideration of Its Nature and Current Implications." *New England Journal of Medicine* 312, no. 5 (1985): 283–89.

"Estriol and Tri-estrogen: Safe Methods of Estrogen Replacement Therapy." *Women's Health Connections,* Apr./May 1994.

Finholm, Valerie. *Hartford Courant,* June 4, 1996.

Finn, Kathleen. "Olive Oil Touted as Breast Cancer Preventive." *Delicious!,* June 1995.

————. "26 Herbs for Better Health." *Delicious!,* July 1996, 30–33, 65–67.

Fioretti, William C. "The Phytochemicals in Dioscorea Provide Support for the Endocrine System." *Proc. 2d Annu. Int. Congr. Alternative Complementary Med.* [Forthcoming].

Follingstad, Alvin H. "Estriol, the Forgotten Estrogen?" *Journal of the American Medical Association* 239, no. 1 (Jan. 2, 1978).

Fuchs, N. K. "Calcium Controversy." *Natural Way,* Apr./May 1995, 12–14.

Fudyma, Janice. *What Do I Take? A Consumer's Guide to Non-Prescription Drugs.* New York: HarperPerennial, 1997.

Garrison, Jayne. "Hormone Therapy: A New Option." *Health,* July/Aug. 1997, 106.

Gittleman, Ann Louise. *Beyond Pritikin*. New York: Bantam, 1988. Rev. ed., 1996.

———. "The Essential Six Female Nutrients." *Healthy Talk,* May 1996, 1–8.

———. *The 40–30–30 Phenomenon*. New Canaan, CT: Keats, 1997.

———. *Super Nutrition for Menopause*. New York: Pocket Books, 1993.

———. *Super Nutrition for Women*. New York: Bantam, 1991.

———. *Your Body Knows Best*. New York: Pocket Books, 1996.

Gladwell, Malcolm. "The Estrogen Question." *New Yorker* (June 9, 1997), 54–61.

Glaspy, John, et al. *J. Natl. Cancer Inst*. (Aug. 1997).

Grady, Denise. "Diet-Diabetes Link Reported." *New York Times,* Feb. 12, 1997.

Graedon, Joe, and Teresa Graedon. *The People's Pharmacy*. Rev. ed. New York: St. Martin's Griffin, 1996.

Haas, Robert. *Permanent Remissions*. New York: Simon & Schuster, 1997.

Hargrove, Joel T., Wayne S. Maxson, and Anne Colston Wentz. "Absorption of Oral Progesterone Is Influenced by Vehicle and Particle Size." *American Journal of Obstetric Gynecology* 161, no. 4 (1989): 948–51.

Hawryluk, Markian. "The Unbeatable Brand: Premarin Topples the Odds Against Off-Patent Success." *Med Ad News* 14, no. 19 (1995).

Herbert, Victor, and Genell Subak-Sharpe, eds. *Total Nutrition*. New York: St. Martin's Press, 1995.

Holt, Stephen. "Phytoestrogens for a Healthier Menopause." *Alternative & Complementary Therapies* 3, no. 3 (June 1997): 187–93.

Hooper, Judith. "Does Menopause Really Begin in Your 30s?" *New Woman,* Aug. 1997.

"Hormone Testing." *Dr. Christiane Northrup's Health Wisdom for Women* 4, no. 7 (July 1997): 1–4.

"Hormone Tests: Blood Versus Saliva." *Women's Health Advocate Newsletter* 3, no. 7 (Sept. 1996): 1–2.

King, Martha. "The Baby Boom Meets Menopause." *Good Housekeeping,* Jan. 1992, 46–50.

Lark, Susan M. *The Estrogen Decision*. Los Altos, CA: Westchester, 1994.

Laudan, Larry. *Danger Ahead: The Risks You Really Face on Life's Highway*. New York: Wiley, 1997.

Laurence, Leslie. "What Women Must Know Before Menopause." *Ladies' Home Journal,* Apr. 1994.

Laux, Marcus, and Christine Conrad. *Natural Woman, Natural Menopause.* New York: HarperCollins, 1997.

Lazarus, Richard S., and Susan Folkman. *Stress, Appraisal, and Coping.* New York: Springer Publishing, 1984.

Lee, John R. *What Your Doctor May Not Tell You About Menopause.* New York: Warner Books, 1996.

Lipson, S., and P. Ellison. "Development of Protocols for the Application of Salivary Steroid Analysis to Field Conditions." *American Journal of Human Biology* 1 (1989): 249–55.

Love, Susan M. *Dr. Susan Love's Hormone Book.* New York: Random House, 1997.

————. "Sometimes Mother Nature Knows Best." *New York Times,* Mar. 20, 1997.

McGowan, Mary P. *Heart Fitness for Life.* New York: Oxford, 1997.

Martin, W. "The Miracle of Evening Primrose Oil." *Townsend Letter for Doctors* (Nov. 1992), 990–92.

Menopause and Perimenopause. Patient Information Series, American Society for Reproductive Medicine, 1992.

Messina, Mark. "Increasing Use of Soy Foods and Their Potential in Cancer Prevention." *Journal of the American Dietetic Association* 91, no. 7 (1991): 836–40.

————. "The Role of Soy Products in Reducing Risk of Cancer." *Journal of the National Cancer Institute* 83, no. 8 (1991): 541–45.

Milligan, Patti Tveit. "Experience the Powerful Benefits of Soy." *Health Counselor,* Aug./Sept. 1997, 57–59.

Morton, M. S. "Determination of Lignans and Isoflavones in Human Female Plasma Following Dietary Supplementation." *Journal of Endocrinology* 142 (1994): 251–59.

Murkies, A. L. "Dietary Flour Supplementation Decreases Post-Menopausal Hot Flashes: Effect of Soy and Wheat." *Maturitas* 21, no. 3 (1995): 189–95.

Nachtigall, Lila E. "Too Young for Hot Flashes?" *Ladies' Home Journal,* July 1996, 110–14.

Northrup, Christiane. *Women's Bodies, Women's Wisdom.* New York: Bantam, 1994.

Ornish, Dean. *Eat More, Weigh Less.* New York: HarperCollins, 1993.

Pelton, Ross, and Lee Overholser. *Revolution in Cancer Therapy.* New York: Fireside, 1994.

Raloff, J. "Hormone Therapy: Issues of the Heart." *Science News* 151 (Mar. 8, 1997): 140.

Rose, David P. *American Journal of Clinical Nutrition* 54 (1991): 520.

Rosenblatt, Robert A. "U.S. Agency Sounds Alarm About 'Miracle' Hormones." *Los Angeles Times,* Apr. 28, 1997.

Rosenfeld, Isadore. "Health Report." *Vogue,* Apr. 1997.

Ryan, George. *Reclaiming Male Sexuality.* New York: Evans, 1997.

Salmeron, Jorge, et al. "Dietary Fiber, Glycemic Load, and Risk of Non-Insulin-Dependent Diabetes Mellitus in Women." *Journal of the American Medical Association* 277, no. 6 (Feb. 12, 1997): 472–77.

Sathyamoorthy, Neerja. "Stimulation of PS2 Expression by Diet-Derived Compounds." *Cancer Res.* 54 (1994): 957–61.

Schofield, Lisa R. "A Balancing Act." *Whole Foods,* July 1997, 21–36.

Sears, Barry. *The Zone.* New York: ReganBooks, 1995.

Shandler, Nina. *Estrogen: The Natural Way.* New York: Villard, 1997.

Sinatra, Stephen S. *Optimum Health.* New York: Bantam, 1997.

"Soybeans Seem to Ease Menopause, Study Shows." *San Francisco Examiner,* Nov. 11, 1996.

Stanford, Janet L., et al. "Combined Estrogen and Progestin Hormone Replacement Therapy in Relation to Risk of Breast Cancer in Middle-Aged Women." *Journal of the American Medical Association* 274 (1995): 137–43.

Stolberg, Sheryl Gay. "Brand-New Recipe for Healthy Bones Adds More Calcium." *New York Times,* Aug. 14, 1997.

Sullivan, Karen, and C. Norman Shealy, eds. *The Complete Family Guide to Natural Home Remedies.* Rockport, MA: Element, 1997.

Upton, Arthur C., and Eden Graber, eds. *Staying Healthy in a Risky Environment: The New York University Medical Center Family Guide.* New York: Simon & Schuster, 1993.

Vliet, Elizabeth Lee. *Screaming to Be Heard.* New York: Evans, 1995.

Vozoff, Kate. "How to Handle the Menopause 'Unmentionable.'" *Townsend Letter for Doctors & Patients,* July 1996, 70–72.

Wallace, Edward C. "Homeopathy: Help for Hot Flashes." *Delicious!,* Oct. 1996, 32–35.

Warga, Claire Landsberg. "Estrogen and the Brain." *New York,* Aug. 11, 1997, 26–31.

Watts, David L. "Premenstrual Impact of Zinc and Copper." *Natural Lifestyling,* Dec. 1993.

Watts, David L. *Trace Elements and Other Essential Nutrients.* Dallas: Trace Elements, 1995.

Winslow, Ron. "Scientists See Promise in New Estrogen Drug." *Wall Street Journal,* Aug. 20, 1997.

"Women's Health: A Special Section." *New York Times,* June 22, 1997.

Wright, Jonathan V., and John Morgenthaler. *Natural Hormone Replacement.* Petaluma, CA: Smart Publications, 1997.

Writing Group for the PEPI Trial. "Effects of Estrogen or Estrogen/Progestin Regimens on Heart Disease Risk Factors in Postmenopausal Women." *Journal of the American Medical Association* 273 (1995): 199–208.

Resources

General Information

For information about perimenopause, write to:

Association of Reproductive Health Professionals
2401 Pennsylvania Avenue, NW, Suite 350
Washington, DC 20037–1718

American Menopause Foundation, Inc.
The Empire State Building
350 Fifth Avenue, Suite 2822
New York, NY 10118
212–714–2398

The American Menopause Foundation is the only independent, not-for-profit organization dedicated to providing support and assistance on all issues concerning the change of life. The network of volunteer support groups serves as a resource for women, families, organizations, and corporations. The foundation's newsletter, literature, and educational programs provide the latest information on scientific research and other pertinent facts.

Power Surge
Internet address:
http://members.aol.com/dearest/intro.htm

Power Surge is a support network and online community for women in varying stages of menopause. Its purpose is to provide information and encourage discourse, enabling every woman to educate herself as to the best method of treatment for her. Celebrated guest authors, physicians, naturopaths, psychotherapists, and nutritionists join in online conferences on a weekly basis.

DHEA Testing

The following laboratory provides a 24-hour urine test to measure DHEA and other steroid hormones.

Meridian Valley Clinical Laboratories
515 West Harrison
Kent, WA 98032
800-234-6825

Education

American Academy of Nutrition
1200 Kenesaw
Knoxville, TN 37919–7736
800–290–4226

The American Academy of Nutrition offers more than twenty nutrition home-study courses as well as a recently developed associate-of-science degree program in applied nutrition. The academy is accredited by the U.S. Department of Education's Distance Education Training Council. I recommend the academy's courses for anyone wishing to become more knowledgeable about such subjects as nutritional counseling, sports nutrition, weight management, and female health concerns.

Newsletter

Dr. Christiane Northrup's monthly newsletter covers many aspects of women's health and natural treatments. $39.95 per year.

Dr. Christiane Northrup's Health Wisdom for Women
7811 Montrose Road
Potomac, MD 20854
800–804–0935

Organics

You can learn about organic food and organic farming from the follow-ing nonprofit organizations.

Organic Trade Association
413-774-7511

Organic Farming Research Foundation
408-426-6606

The Land Institute
913-823-5376

Community Alliance with Family Farmers
916-756-8518

Referrals

For a referral to a medical doctor or osteopath who is knowledgeable in the use of natural hormone replacement, you can contact:

The American College for Advancement in Medicine (ACAM)
23121 Verdug Drive, Suite 204
Laguna Hills, CA 92653
800-532-3688

Naturopathic physicians are licensed in the following states: Alaska, Arizona, Connecticut, Hawaii, Maine, Montana, New Hampshire, Ore-gon, Utah, Vermont, Washington, and the District of Columbia. For a referral to a naturopathic physician who can guide you with natural hor-mone therapy, you can contact:

The American Association of Naturopathic Physicians
2366 East Lake Avenue, Suite 322
Seattle, WA 98102
206-328-8510

Salivary Hormone Testing

For information about a saliva test for hormone levels and to order a prepaid mailer for it:

Aeron LifeCycles
1933 Davis Street, Suite 310
San Leandro, CA 94577
800–631–7900
http://www.aeron.com.

Diagnos-Techs, Inc.
6620 S. 192nd Pl., J–104
Kent, WA 98032
800–878–3787

Specialty Supplements, Products, and Books

Uni Key Health Systems
P.O. Box 7168
Bozeman, MT 59771
800–888–4353

Uni Key Health Systems has distributed supplements to my own clients and readers for over five years. They offer a female copper-free multiple and other formulas, such as their adrenal gland support. The Tru-Temperature Health System and the Doulton water filter can be ordered. Ask for a brochure of all the latest products. If you can't find my books in the bookstore, Uni Key can send them to you directly.

Water

The National Resources Defense Council (NRDC) sells three publications on drinking water. For information, contact:

NRDC Information
40 West 20th Street
New York, NY 10011
212-727-2700

Environmental Protection Agency Safe Drinking Water Hot Line
800-426-4791

To find a local lab to have your drinking water tested, look under "Laboratories, Testing" in your phone book. If there are none, you can contact these mail-order water-testing laboratories:

National Testing Laboratories, Inc.
6555 Wilson Mills Road
Cleveland, OH 44143
800-458-3330

Suburban Water Testing Laboratories, Inc.
4600 Kutztown Road
Temple, PA 19560
800-433-6595

Health Pharmacies

Many of us may remember when a pharmacist actually combined ingredients to create our medicine, carefully measuring and mixing the ingredients to the doctor's order and making a remedy specifically for us. Nowadays, when you take your prescription to the pharmacy, they merely fill the bottle with a ready-made pill to be used by everyone.

While it's true that most pharmacies no longer practice compounding of prescriptions on a personal basis, I am delighted to provide a list of health pharmacies that do so. Some even provide a referral listing of doctors who use natural hormone remedies for prescriptions. However, if you prefer to locate a health pharmacy closer to home, you can call the International Academy of Compounding Pharmacists in Sugarland,

Texas (713–933–8400 or 800–927–4227). They will assist you in locating a local pharmacy that specializes in compounding natural prescriptions.
    Organized by state in alphabetical order:

Wellness Health &
  Pharmaceuticals
2800 South 18th Street
Birmingham, AL 35209
800–227–2627

Mountain View Pharmacy
10565 North Tatum Blvd.,
Suite B118
Paradise Valley, AZ 85253
602–948–7065

Artesia Pharmacy
18550 South Pioneer Blvd.
Artesia, CA 90701
800–851–7900

Oaks Pharmacy
4940 Van Nuys Blvd.
Sherman Oaks, CA 91403
818–990–3784

Doc's Pharmacy
112 La Casa Via, Suite 100
Walnut Creek, CA 94598
510–939–6311

Eddie's Pharmacy
8500 Melrose Avenue
West Hollywood, CA 90069
310–358–2400

College Pharmacy
833 North Tejon Street
Colorado Springs, CO 80903
800–888–9358

    The College Pharmacy in Colorado Springs is probably the most complete pharmacy specializing in natural hormone replacement therapy. They also stock antiaging hormones and dermatological formulas and injectables. Consulting pharmacist Pete Heuseman, at extension 4116, will be glad to answer your questions.

Belmar Pharmacy
8015 W. Alameda Avenue,
Suite 100
Lake Wood, CO 80226

Trumarx Drugs
501 Gordon Avenue
Thomasville, GA 31792
800–552–9997

Professional Arts Pharmacy
1101 North Rolling Road
Baltimore, MD 21225
800–832–9285

Diplomat Pharmacy
3426 Flushing Road
Flint, MI 48504
810–732–8720

Bajamar Women's Health Care
9609 Dielman Rock Island
St. Louis, MO 63132

The Apothecary
35 Main Street
Keene, NH 03431
603-357-0200

Wedgewood Village Pharmacy
373 K Egg Harbor Road
Sewell, NJ 08080
609-589-4200

Apthorp Pharmacy
2201 Broadway
New York, NY 10024
212-877-3480

Hospital Discount Pharmacy
104 South Bryant
Edmonds, OK 73034
405-348-1677

Delk Pharmacy
1602 Hatcher Lane
Columbia, TN 38401
616-388-3952

The Medicine Shoppe
1567 North Eastman Road
Kingsport, TN 37664
423-245-1022

Apothecure
13720 Midway Road, Suite 109
Dallas, TX 75244
800-969-6601

Greenpark Pharmacy
7515 South Main
Houston, TX 77030
713-795-5812

Medical Center Pharmacy
10721 Main Street
Fairfax, VA 22030
800-723-9160

Belgrove Pharmacy
1535 116th Avenue NE
Bellevue, WA 98004
800-446-2123

Madison Pharmacy Associates
429 Gammon Place
P.O. Box 9641
Madison, WI 53715
800-558-7046

**Women's International
  Pharmacy**
5708 Monona Drive
Madison, WI 53716-3152
800-279-5708

List of Products Recommended

Adrenal Formula, from Uni Key
Health Systems
Balance Bar
Bragg Liquid Aminos
Clorox
Creme de la Femme, from Uni Key
Health Systems
Doulton Ceramic Water Filter
EasySoy, from Carlson
Eskimo 3, from Cardinova
Featherweight baking powder
Flax Oil Hi Lignan, from
Barlean's
Friendship cottage cheese
Glycemic Balance by Jarrow
Formulas

Gy-Na-Tren, from Natren
Iso-Gen, from Bio Nutritional
Formulas
Key-E ointment or suppositories,
from Carlson
Kraft Breakstone 2 percent cottage
cheese
MAG-200 tablets, from Optimox
Magnesium Forte, from Uni Key
Health Systems
MaxEPA, from Solgar
Meno-Fem, from Prevail
Mori-Nu tofu
Old Home cottage cheese
Omega-3 fish oil concentrate,
from Dale Alexander

Omega Twin Hi Lignan, from
Barlean's
Phyto-EST, from BioTherapies
Pro-Estron, from Neutraceutics
Corporation
Rejuvex
Remifemin, from Enzymatic
Therapy
Roma, Bambu, and Cafix drinks
Royal Jelly, from Bee-Alive
Saliva tests from Aeron LifeCycles
Super Omega–3, Norwegian
salmon oil, and evening
primrose oil, from Carlson
The Essential Woman oil, from
Barlean's Organic Oils
Uni Key Female Multiple, from
Uni Key Health Systems
Vegetable Protein from Naturade
Vitex
Whey to Go, from Solgar
White Wave, an organic tofu
Yeast-Guard vaginal suppository

Equilibrium, from Equilibrium
Lab
Femme Naturale, from Sarati
International
NatraGest, from Broadmoore
Labs
OstaDerm, from Bezwecken
PhytoGest, from Karuna
Corp.
Pro-Alo, from HealthWatchers
Pro-G, from TriMedica
Pro-Gest, from Professional &
Technical Services
ProBalance, from Springboard
Progonal, from Bezwecken

Foods
(in recipe chapter)

AK-Mak crackers
Health Valley whole-wheat
crackers
Stevita, stevia
Real salt
Ryvita breads
Spectrum Lite mayonnaise
Wasa breads
Westbrae rice wafers

Creams

Angel Care, from Angel Care
Bio Balance, from Garon
Pharmaceuticals

Index

241